Modern Infectious
Disease Epidemiology

The front cover shows the two nautical signal flags, Q and L, which, when hoisted together, signify that a ship has infectious disease on board.

Modern Infectious Disease Epidemiology

Second edition

By

Johan Giesecke
Professor of Infectious Disease Epidemiology

Karolinska Institute,
Stockholm
Sweden

ARNOLD

A member of the Hodder Headline Group
LONDON • NEW YORK • NEW DELHI

First published in Great Britain in 1994
Second edition published in 2002 by
Arnold, a member of the Hodder Headline Group,
338 Euston Road, London NW1 3BH

Distributed in the USA by
Oxford University Press Inc.,
198 Madison Avenue, New York NY10016
Oxford is a registered trademark of Oxford University Press

http://www.arnoldpublishers.com

British Library Cataloguing in Publication Data
A catalogue record for this book is available from the British Library

Library of Congress Cataloging-in-Publication Data
A catalog record for this book is available from the Library of Congress

ISBN 0 340 76423 6

2 3 4 5 6 7 8 9 10

Publisher: Georgina Bentliff
Production Editor: Jasmine Brown
Production Controller: Martin Kerans
Cover Design: Terry Griffiths

Typeset in 9½/14pt Sabon by Phoenix Photosetting, Chatham, Kent
Printed and bound in Great Britain by the MPG Books Ltd, Bodmin, Cornwall

What do you think about this book? Or any other Arnold title?
Please send your comments to feedback.arnold@hodder.co.uk

To Kajsa and the Pie Bunch

Contents

Contents

Preface to the second edition

The reception of this book during the seven years since it was published has exceeded my expectations. Whilst it may not have caused any overturning of booksellers' stands (which my brother, who has experience of the publishing business, uses as a measure of a book's success), a number of people I had never met before have come up to me and told me that they liked it.

Since finishing the first edition, I spent a year and a half as a clinician, but it is now five years since I saw a real patient, and I doubt if I ever will again (except for neighbours and next-of-kin). This is a drawback for an epidemiologist, since I feel that close contact with clinical work helps one to keep one's perspective. However, as someone once said, there are only two musts in life: 'you must choose, and you must die', and my present work precludes any clinical activity. But one never knows, a major advantage of medical training is the lingering possibility of going back to work with patients. And I still nurture the dream of training in intensive care to the point where I could remain calm and efficient when people are on the brink of dying all around me.

The need for a second edition has been evident for a long time. There were some blatant errors in the first edition, and I am particularly grateful to Professor Jonathan Freeman at the Harvard School of Public Health for pointing several of them out to me. I also thank colleagues and students for constructive comments along the way.

All of the chapters have been revised, some quite extensively, and mostly through the addition of new thoughts or new examples. The short chapter on descriptive epidemiology is new, and the last chapter now uses variant CJD as well as AIDS to illustrate the full spectrum of methodological problems. Several readers have missed suggestions for further reading, so I have added a personal list at the end.

One piece of advice to the reader who is considering becoming an author. Never agree with your publisher to revise a book. It is much more work than it seems. However, if it has made the book more accessible and instructive, it has been worthwhile.

Johan Giesecke
Geneva and Stockholm, 2001

Preface to the first edition

In many ways this is the book that I myself would have liked to read some five years ago, when I first became interested in the epidemiology of infectious diseases. At that time I had been working as an infectious disease physician for several years, and I was becoming particularly curious about the epidemiology of AIDS. How infectious was this disease really? How long did it take from someone becoming infected with HIV until he or she developed AIDS? Why did the epidemic assume such seemingly disparate shapes in different countries and different subpopulations?

When I started to look into the basic literature on epidemiology, I found few books that addressed the issues in the way that I wanted them to be addressed. The authors generally assumed a different perspective, and the examples given in the text had little to do with situations or diseases with which I felt familiar. Conversely, I found that books on the epidemiology of infectious diseases generally dealt more with characteristics of the individual diseases, and that they seldom addressed the methodological and conceptual problems of infectious disease epidemiology *per se*.

Also, quite early in research on AIDS many authors perceived and commented upon the importance of contact patterns for the development of the epidemic. Who meets whom in the population? Few basic textbooks in epidemiology deal with contact patterns in a constructive way, and yet they are crucial to the epidemiology of almost all infectious diseases.

Nevertheless, I slowly worked my way through the literature, often having to re-interpret what I had just read to conform with my views and problems. At some time during those years, I had the idea of writing a book better tailored to the epidemiology of infectious diseases. During the academic year 1991–92, I received a scholarship from the Swedish Medical Research Council to learn epidemiology properly at the London School of Hygiene and Tropical Medicine, and during that year the structure of this book began to take shape. The contents – especially as regards collection of illustrative examples from published studies – were completed during my second year at the School, when I somewhat unexpectedly was offered a post as Senior Lecturer in epidemiology for a year. Now, however, I am returning to Sweden, for some time at least, because I believe that any physician who wants to do relevant work in epidemiology has to maintain a strong contact with his or her clinical roots. Without such bonds with the starting place of all epidemiology, one is in peril of losing one's perspective and sense of direction.

Thanks are due to my friend Professor Gian-Paolo Scalia-Tomba at the Department of Statistics of the University La Sapienza in Rome for having revised and commented on all the statistical parts of the book, making sure that my naïve attitude to statistics did not become too simplified. I am also grateful to Dr Elizabeth Miller of the Communicable Diseases Surveillance Centre in London for supplying me with the data for the graph on measles incidence in England and Wales in Chapter 10. Furthermore, I want to thank my publishers, Edward Arnold, and in particular Louise Cook, for the rapid decision to publish and a very supportive attitude. Finally, although for reasons outside our control it has not been possible for him to read the manuscript of this book, I have enjoyed immensely all the stimulating discussions with my boss and friend, Professor Paul Fine, in which he has willingly shared his profound knowledge about the epidemiology of infectious diseases.

When writing this book I have tried to cast my own mind back five years, assuming the knowledge, ideas and misconceptions I had when I started to study epidemiology, and thus trying to write for a reader who is at a similar level now. It is always hard to remember why something was so difficult to understand at first and what the obstacles were. Some of the ideas and examples may not be new to those who already share my fascination with the multifaceted and intellectually challenging field of infectious disease epidemiology, but I hope that other aspects as well as the general structure of this book will prove interesting to them. I also hope that I have been able to transmit some of this fascination to such readers as have not yet seen the light of infectious disease epidemiology.

Johan Giesecke
London and Stockholm, 1994

Introduction

This book has been written for people with an interest in infectious diseases who want to learn more about epidemiology. It does not assume any specialist knowledge of infectious disease medicine or microbiology, certainly no more than most practising physicians would have.

However, I have always maintained that an infectious disease perspective is a good place to start learning epidemiology in general, since many of the concepts become clearer and more intuitive when explained with examples about infections. This may be especially true for clinicians who want to learn more about epidemiology. One problem I have found with many otherwise excellent introductory texts on epidemiology is that they present the subject more from a public health perspective than from a clinical view point, and this tends to make the concepts, terminology and even examples somewhat unfamiliar to someone with a clinical background.

The book is loosely divided into two parts. The first chapter begins with some philosophizing about the quintessence of infectious diseases epidemiology. It is followed by a chapter that defines the central terms of this branch of science, and you may well want to skip this at first, only to return to it when the terms appear later in the text. Chapters 3 to 10 then explain concepts and methods that are basic to all branches of epidemiology, such as risk, rate, odds, confounding, bias, sensitivity, specificity and different types of epidemiological studies. Some basic statistical procedures are also covered. Similar material can be found in other books on epidemiology, the difference being that the perspective here is at times somewhat personal and the illustrative examples, both published and invented, all concern infectious diseases.

The second part of the book applies the tools learned in the first part to the specific issues of infectious disease epidemiology, such as outbreaks, surveillance, infectiousness, immunity, seroepidemiology and vaccines. Chapter 11 gives the conceptual background to the discussion in the subsequent chapters, and even if you do not like mathematics you should spend some time trying to familiarize yourself with these ideas because they are central to the understanding of many infectious disease phenomena. This part of the book relies heavily on examples from published studies on infectious diseases. The last chapter uses two diseases with a rather complex epidemiology – AIDS and variant CJD – to recapitulate large parts of what has been covered previously. Some of the chapters in this part may also be of interest to those with previous experience in epidemiology who want to learn more about the specifics of infectious disease epidemiology.

One note of caution should be given. I have tried to keep the style of the book as simple and untechnical as possible. The basic common-sense ideas of epidemiology should not be obscured by difficult jargon. However, from experience I know that some concepts take longer to grasp than others, and some sections may require re-reading once or twice even if the style used in the book makes them seem obvious at first reading.

Another point is that the tables and graphs have been placed in the text exactly where they should be looked at. When I read a scientific article I often skip the tables (which are usually on the next page anyway) just to see what will come next in the text proper. I strongly recommend that you do not do this when reading this book, but instead give yourself time to study the tables and graphs when they appear.

Finally, a disproportionate number of examples in the book come from studies in which I myself have been involved. This is certainly not because they are better than those of other people. It is just that I am familiar with these studies, and for some of the examples I have made use of primary data which have been easily accessible.

Chapter 1
What is special about infectious disease epidemiology?

Some general ideas about epidemiology are discussed and a few reasons are given as to why you should read a book specifically about the epidemiology of infectious diseases.

What is epidemiology and why should one spend time studying it? Most standard definitions of epidemiology mention something like 'the study of diseases and their determinants in populations', which is an adequate if somewhat abstract formulation.

My own practical view is that epidemiology is about putting people into groups. We are all individuals, and no two patients are ever exactly alike. Even the largest forest consists of trees each of which is unique. However, we all have a number of characteristics that group us with other people – we are either male or female, we are of a certain age, we live in a certain area, we have certain dietary habits and behaviours, etc., and we share those characteristics with varying numbers of our fellow human beings. Epidemiology identifies such groups, ignoring the uniqueness of its members, and tries to determine whether this division of people into groups tells us something more than we could have learned by merely observing each person separately. Since epidemiology is a branch of medicine, our interest is usually to describe, analyse or understand patterns of disease in such groups. The most common situation occurs when we find one group of people who are ill with some disease, and another group of individuals who are not. What is the difference between these groups? Is there some characteristic that seems to differ between them?

Epidemiology is thus largely a matter of perspective, and a colleague of mine, who is one of the best clinicians I have met, once said of himself 'I will never be a good epidemiologist – I cannot see the forest, I can only see the trees.' This is a perfectly justifiable position, and medicine needs both types of approach.

At a basic level, epidemiology starts with a description of the cases of a disease. When do they appear and where? What ages are they? Is there any group-defining characteristic that they have in common? Obviously, in such descriptions it is not the individual cases that are of prime interest, but rather the collective pattern of disease that they form. Such straightforward *descriptive epidemiology* almost always reveals interesting patterns that we would not have observed if we had not collected the cases and ordered them in a structured manner. To the inquisitive mind (and unless you had one you would not be reading this book), the question 'why?' pops up immediately. Why were there so many cases in a certain area? Why were there more women than men? Why were there no sick children? Why are there more cases this year than last?

Such questions lead to the next step in the epidemiological analysis. We move on to *analytical epidemiology*, which usually means that we try systematically to compare the group of disease cases with another group of healthy people. We test the clues offered by the descriptive study by searching for differences in characteristics between the ill and the healthy. Did the cases of gastroenteritis eat something that the others did not eat? Did the children who contracted measles go to a different school to those who did not? Is it more common to find evidence of coxsackie virus infection in children with diabetes than in healthy children? Will there be more cases of tuberculosis during the next year in a group of HIV-infected people than in a group who test negative for HIV? If our analytical study has been well designed, and if the clues we are investigating are appropriate, we may find strong support for a certain aetiology, a certain pathological mechanism or a certain source.

The final step is to convert our knowledge about this disease into preventive action. Can hygiene measures be instigated by society? Can we influence people's behaviour so as to reduce their risk of falling ill? Is there any prophylactic treatment? Could a vaccine be developed? Here again, epidemiology might be called upon to evaluate the effects of preventive measures. Did they have the effect on pattern of disease that we had hoped for?

SOME SPECIAL FEATURES

With the exception of vaccination, all of these steps apply equally to non-infectious and infectious disease epidemiology. However, there are two features that are unique to the infectious diseases.

1. *A case may also be a risk factor.*

2. *People may be immune.*

With regard to the first feature, in most non-infectious disease epidemiology the division between the risk factors for disease and the cases themselves is unambiguous. Smoking is a risk factor, and a patient with lung cancer is a case. Radiation is a risk factor, and a patient with leukaemia is a case. High alcohol intake is a risk factor, and a patient with cirrhosis is a case. In all of these examples, the risk factors belong to a completely different category to the cases. A person's risk of developing coronary heart disease is not influenced by his neighbour's myocardial infarction. Nor does intensive treatment of coronary thrombosis patients in hospital reduce the overall rate of new cases of this disease in the population.

However, for influenza, my risk of disease during the coming winter will be greatly affected by the number of influenza patients around, and if many of the people I meet have been vaccinated, my risk of contracting influenza will decrease even if I myself have not been vaccinated. Treatment of a tuberculosis case will dramatically reduce the risk of disease in members of that individual's family. For many of the infectious diseases, someone who is a case will at the same time be a risk factor for disease in other people. Thus the clear distinction between the two categories in the above paragraph becomes blurred. The fact that a case may be a source of disease in others also means that contact patterns in society (who meets whom, how they meet and how often) become very important issues if we want to understand the epidemiology of infectious diseases.

Some scientists working in non-infectious disease epidemiology become annoyed when I point out to them that they are dealing with a simplified version of the science, namely one in which transmission of disease between cases does not have to be accounted for.

The second feature, namely immunity, is also unique to infectious diseases. Someone who has had measles will never get it again, even if he strolls through ward after ward of measles patients. For most non-infectious risk factors, such as toxins or radiation, there will be levels at which everyone exposed will fall ill. (It could be argued that some kind of *resistance* to such risks also exists. Why do some people remain healthy after having smoked two packets of cigarettes a day for 50 years? However, very little is known about this type of resistance.)

These two points represent the major differences between the two branches of epidemiology, but there are a few more.

3. A case may be a source without being recognized as a case.

By this I mean that asymptomatic or subclinical infections play an important role in the epidemiology of many infectious diseases. Ignorance of their existence would make many outbreaks and transmission chains inexplicable.

4. There is sometimes a need for urgency.

Most current non-infectious disease epidemiology is concerned with environmental and behavioural risk factors for disease. Investigations are often large-scale and lengthy, and their results may enter into public health programmes that often take years to implement. With outbreaks of infectious diseases, the time-frame is sometimes closer to hours or days before some preventive action has to be decided on. This may give little time for elaborate analyses.

5. *Preventive measures (usually) have a good scientific basis.*

Much is known about the bacteria, viruses and other parasites that cause disease, about their transmission, and about how they should be stopped, even if this knowledge may not always have the desired public health impact. Someone who, like myself, has been observing the 30-year debate on the dangers of cholesterol, or the discussion about what causes asthma in children, from the sidelines may easily feel content to be in the field of infectious diseases. With some exaggeration, one could say that infectious disease epidemiology is largely concerned with the investigation of preventive factors, whereas non-infectious disease epidemiology is still struggling with risk factors.

Some authors denote what I have termed 'non-infectious' above as 'chronic' disease epidemiology, implying among other things cancer and cardiovascular disease. This is not very accurate, since several of the infectious diseases are just as chronic as many of the non-infectious ones.

EPIDEMIOLOGY AND DIAGNOSIS

When dealing with patients with infectious diseases we use epidemiology all the time, without even thinking about it. When taking a patient history, we ask questions like the following.

- Does anyone else in the family cough?

- How long after the dinner did you start to feel sick?

- Have you been to the tropics?

- How long is it since his brother had a rash?

The answers to all of these questions aid our diagnosis. Compare this with the usefulness of the question 'Do you know of any neighbour with similar chest pain?' for deciding whether or not the patient in front of us has a myocardial infarction. Or how useful would the question 'Did her sister break her ankle recently?' be in helping to determine whether the patient has a fracture or just a strained ligament?

Our almost subconscious knowledge of incubation times, transmission routes, geographical risk zones, etc. is an important tool in diagnosis, but few clinicians I have met seem to realize to what extent they are using epidemiological facts when they interview a patient in the emergency room or the clinic.

SUMMARY

Most aspects of infectious disease epidemiology are similar to those of non-infectious disease epidemiology. The terminology, concepts and analysis are basically the same. However, the five special features outlined above, and especially the added complication that disease can spread from one case to another, not only makes this branch of epidemiology much more intellectually challenging, but it also increases the risk of scientific mistakes. Those who want to devote some serious effort to the study of infectious diseases would do well to consider those special aspects.

Chapter 2
Definitions

This chapter deals with a number of the definitions and concepts necessary for understanding the literature on infectious disease epidemiology.

Every self-respecting branch of science needs to have its own language and concepts. Sometimes it borrows words that have certain connotations in everyday language and gives them a strict definition with a slightly different meaning. Philosophy, sociology and psychiatry contain a number of such examples, but even within somatic medicine they are not uncommon. For example, a 'positive test result' can mean something quite different to the doctor and to the layman, and 'stress' now denotes a well-defined response of the neuroendocrine system, and not an everyday situation of significant concern.

The purpose of such words is not to deter the novice, but rather to lay a foundation for precise communication. The words of everyday language often have an ambiguity that creates misunderstandings. Some examples are listed below.

1. What do we mean by saying that a disease is common? Do we mean that many have it, or that many will get it?

2. If we say that 'the mortality in disease X is high', do we mean that X is a common cause of death, or that a large proportion of those who contract X will die?

3. What does 'infected' mean? Does it mean that a person is ill, or that they soon will be?

4. If we state that 'the risk of becoming infected with Y is high', do we mean that there is a high probability of meeting someone with Y, or that the risk of transmission is high once we meet someone who demonstrably has Y?

SOME GENERAL DEFINITIONS

Incidence

Incidence is defined as the number of individuals who fall ill with a certain disease during a defined time period, divided by the total population. If the time period is not stated, it is usually assumed to be one year. Thus the statement that 'the incidence of hepatitis B in Sweden is about 2 per 100 000' means that for every 100 000 inhabitants in Sweden, some two individuals contract hepatitis B each year. For common diseases, the incidence may be expressed as a percentage or 'per 1000 population', while for rare diseases a greater denominator is used – for example, 'the annual incidence of Creutzfeldt–Jakob's disease in most Western countries seems to lie between 1 and 2 per 1 million inhabitants'.

In most instances, incidence is calculated from clinical cases, but by following people with serological tests it is possible to detect the subclinical cases, and thus to obtain an incidence figure for the true number of infections.

If incidence is measured over a longer time period, it is often replaced by the term *cumulative incidence*. If we find that 40% of 5-year-olds have antibodies to varicella virus, we can say that the cumulative incidence during the first 5 years of life is 40%, but we do not know exactly how the incidence has varied over these years.

Prevalence

The prevalence of a disease is the number of people who have that disease at a specific time, divided by the total population. For example, 'The prevalence of HIV infection in several African countries is above 20 per 100 population.'

A person who falls ill adds 1 to the incidence of the disease. He will also add 1 to the prevalence for the duration of his disease, until he either recovers or dies. If the average daily incidence of a disease is I and the average duration is D days, then the average prevalence P will be:

$$P = I \times D$$

Alternatively, expressed in words, 'prevalence is the product of incidence and duration'. Most infectious diseases have such a rapid course that 'prevalence' becomes a rather uninteresting measure. Even disregarding the fact that it would be very difficult to count every individual who had, say, campylobacter diarrhoea in a country on any single day, the seasonal variations are so large as to render prevalence figures rather meaningless. The prevalence of influenza A infection in England can be several per cent in January for certain years, but zero in July.

For chronic or protracted infections, matters become somewhat different. Prevalence figures can be very interesting for hepatitis B carriage, chlamydia infection or HIV infection. For such diseases, the prevalence gives some indication of the risk of exposure to others in the population. For example, if we assume that a person with acute hepatitis B is infectious over a period of 2 months, then the prevalence of individuals who are infectious with hepatitis B at the present time will be equal to the number of carriers plus one-sixth of the yearly incidence (assuming an even incidence over the year and also including subclinical infections).

When using serology to determine the percentage of a population that shows markers of having had a disease, we often use the term *seroprevalence*. One could argue that this is stretching the term, and that the proportion of a population with markers is really a measure of the cumulative incidence, but it would be cumbersome to put *sero-* in front of that term.

Denominator

The above two definitions highlight a central concept in epidemiology, that when comparing incidence (or prevalence) between two groups one must take into account the size of the groups – the denominator. The incidence of meningococcal meningitis in Sweden is about 1 per 100 000 inhabitants per year, whereas in Denmark it is considerably higher. Since the population of Denmark is about half that of Sweden, the same number of meningitis cases in both countries during a year would mean that the Danish incidence is about twice as high. Three cases of tuberculosis in a small town would give a high local incidence for that town, but may not affect the figure for national incidence very much. Figures given for various events and conditions in epidemiology should always be divided by the number of individuals in the population under consideration.

There is some confusion in the epidemiological literature here. Especially in older texts, incidence and prevalence were taken to be the actual number of cases, regardless of the denominator. The corresponding measures divided by their denominators were then usually called the *incidence rate* and *prevalence rate*. I would discourage the use of these terms, and maintain that figures for incidence and prevalence should only be given with a denominator as above. Such practice encourages awareness of the crucial denominator concept in our epidemiological thinking. Sometimes, this denominator might be implicit. For example, 'The incidence of reported salmonella in Sweden in 2000 was 4848' implicitly means 'per 8.9 million population', and is thus less satisfactory, since not everyone will know the population of Sweden offhand.

If the denominator cannot even be defined, you should not use the word 'incidence' at all. Thus the statement 'the incidence of gonorrhoea among gay men in London in 1999 was X' is meaningless, since no one would know the denominator. The correct statement would be 'there were X cases of gonorrhoea among gay men in London in 1999'.

In real life you will find that practice varies as to whether figures for incidence and prevalence have already been divided by a denominator or not, but it is usually clear from the content which definition is being used. I also believe that practice is gradually moving towards the definitions that I provided above.

Population at risk

National statistics on infectious diseases usually give the annual incidence per 100 000 inhabitants, with the population counted at mid-year. In other instances it may be less evident what the denominator should be.

For diseases that could only affect one of the sexes, such as orchitis or salpingitis, the denominator should just include the number of individuals of the respective sex in the population. If the incidence of a disease is expressed by age group, the denominator should be the number of individuals in each age group in the population. This is important, since the size of different age groups may vary considerably.

One recurrent issue in infectious disease epidemiology is whether the incidence for diseases that lead to immunity should have the total population, or just those who have not yet contracted the disease, in the denominator. Since the proportion who are immune is often not known, the former is generally used, but if one does know how many have already had the disease, one should divide by the number of individuals who are still susceptible.

In general, one should strive to include only those who *could* get the disease in the denominator (i.e. the *population at risk*).

Case fatality rate or lethality

The term 'case fatality rate' is almost exclusively used in infectious disease epidemiology, whilst people outside our field tend to use the term 'lethality' (or inversely the 'rate of survival', which has a more positive ring to it). They both mean the same thing, namely the proportion of people who will die of a certain disease out of those who contract it. For acute infections, one needs some time limit from the start of the illness, and the case fatality rate for measles is thus often measured as those who die within 4–6 weeks after the rash appears.

Figures for the case fatality rate are largely dependent on how many of the milder cases escape diagnosis. The very high figures initially cited for the case fatality rate in haemorrhagic fevers, such as Lassa fever, were probably largely explained by the fact that many of the more benign cases remained undetected by the local health authorities.

Mortality

This measure indicates what proportion of the entire population die from the disease each year.

In Western Europe a disease such as rabies has a high case fatality rate but low mortality. All of those infected die, but the number of deaths is only a few per year. Conversely, influenza A has a low case fatality rate (most cases survive) but may carry a high mortality. During an influenza epidemic the percentage of all deaths in the country that are due to influenza can be seen to rise markedly. Since influenza is responsible for a sizeable proportion of all deaths during an epidemic, mortality from all other causes may show a slight temporary decrease.

People frequently talk about 'mortality' when they mean 'case fatality rate'.

DEFINITIONS USED IN INFECTIOUS DISEASE EPIDEMIOLOGY

There are a number of definitions that are chiefly or only used in infectious disease epidemiology. The first concerns the subject itself. What exactly does the term 'infectious diseases' encompass?

One could make a distinction such as the following.

- Infectious diseases – all diseases caused by micro-organisms.

- Communicable diseases – diseases that can be transmitted from one infected person to another, directly or indirectly.

- Transmissible diseases – diseases that can be transmitted from one person to another by 'unnatural' routes.

In the above, each group is a subset of the previous one.

Legionnaire's disease and tetanus are examples of diseases that are infectious but not communicable. Measles, influenza and shigellosis are all both infectious and communicable. Creutzfeldt–Jacob's disease can be passed from one patient to the next via neurosurgical instruments or corneal transplants, neither of which is a 'natural' route, and it is thus a transmissible disease. (In this context, it is interesting to note the term 'sexually transmitted disease' (STD), which hints at an underlying moralistic conception that sexual contact is a non-natural transmission route. 'Sexually communicable disease' (SCD) would be a better term than STD.)

In this book we shall not make any distinction between *infectious* and *communicable* diseases. The John M. Last *Dictionary of Epidemiology* defines infectious disease as follows:[1]

> An illness due to a specific infectious agent or its toxic products that arises through transmission of that agent or its products from an infected person, animal or reservoir to a susceptible host, either directly or indirectly through an intermediate plant or animal host, vector or the inanimate environment.

Contagious disease is a slightly obsolete term, but if used nowadays it usually means 'highly infectious'.

We shall now go on to discuss several other important definitions.

Someone who has met with an infectious agent in a way that we know from experience may cause disease has been *exposed*. You will immediately notice that this definition is circular, since our concept of exposure will rely on our current biological knowledge of transmission mechanisms. Someone who passes a patient with a salmonella infection in a corridor has not been exposed to salmonella. However, a child who has been playing in the same room as another child with pertussis has been exposed to whooping cough.

If the infectious agent manages to get a foothold in the exposed person, that individual becomes *infected*. Sometimes this will lead to changes that are clinically evident or can be assessed by laboratory tests. The most obvious outcome is that he falls ill (i.e. has a *clinical infection*). Frequently the infected person will not display any symptoms, but can be shown serologically to have reacted to the infectious agent. He has then had a *subclinical* (or *asymptomatic*) *infection*.

Both types of infection can lead to a *carrier* state for some diseases. A carrier harbours the pathogen, and is able to transmit it, but shows no clinical signs of infection. Such a state may be prolonged compared to the acute infection. Examples include hepatitis B and salmonella infections.

The different outcomes of exposure to an infectious agent are shown in Figure 2.1.

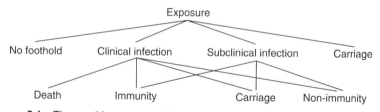

Figure 2.1   The possible outcomes of exposure to an infectious agent.

For a few bacteria a somewhat different carrier state is also possible. The best example is that of staphylococci, which a person might carry on their skin or in their nose and transmit to others. In this carrier state the person is not really infected with the bacteria, but rather they are locally *colonized*.

The two different carrier states are not identical, and should really have two different names.

The role played by subclinical infections and carrier states in the spread of infectious diseases constitutes an important part of modern infectious disease epidemiology, and is one of the phenomena whereby this branch of epidemiology most clearly displays its distinctive traits.

Someone who has contracted an infection (clinical or subclinical) with a certain pathogen – or who has been vaccinated against it – so that he shows no clinical signs of infection on renewed exposure to this pathogen, is said to be *immune*. However, it is sometimes possible to show by laboratory methods that an already immune person has reacted to the exposure with an increased antibody titre, and this is called a *natural booster*. Those who are not immune to a disease, and who are thus potentially infected by an exposure, are said to be *susceptible*.

An important factor that determines the risk of becoming infected is the *dose* (i.e. the actual number of micro-organisms that are attacking the person). Whereas a low number of bacteria or virus particles may be fended off directly by the body, a massive dose is almost certain to lead to infection in a susceptible individual.

What is a case?

Much of routine infectious disease epidemiology relies on reports of notifiable diseases. Using such figures, cases may be compared over time or between regions and countries. The above graph of possible outcomes following exposure makes it clear that the definition of a case is far from simple.

To be registered as a case in the classical sense, the following criteria have to be met.

1. The patient:

    - has to experience symptoms from the infection; and

    - has to be ill enough to seek medical care or advice.

2. The physician:

    - has to suspect the correct diagnosis; and

    - (usually) has to send a sample to the laboratory.

3. The tests in the laboratory:

    - must come out positive; and

4. The case must be reported.

Finally, the case must be filed correctly by some central agency.

It is obvious that the number of cases included in regional/national statistics will underestimate the true number of infections to varying degrees for different diseases.

The increasing use of laboratory methods to ascertain subclinical diseases complicates the picture even further. For example, if we start a large screening programme for genital chlamydia infection (which is often asymptomatic), the number of reported chlamydia cases will rise sharply, which might give the impression of a sudden epidemic. Furthermore, for some diseases that are mainly diagnosed by serology, such as hepatitis B and syphilis, there can be ambiguity as to whether the patient represents a new case or just has markers of an old infection, and even if they can be shown just to have markers of an old infection, they must still have been a case at some point between conception and the present.

Attack rate

This is defined as the proportion of individuals who are exposed to an infectious agent who become (clinically) ill. Obviously any calculation of the attack rate will depend on how accurately exposure and disease are measured. If some of the individuals who were exposed were not counted, the calculated attack rate would be too high, and if instead some of the cases were missed, the attack rate would appear too low. Moreover, for most calculations of attack rate one would want to exclude individuals who were exposed and who were already immune to the disease (i.e. only include the population at risk).

Primary/secondary cases

For infections that are spread from person to person, the individual who brings the disease into a population (where the population can be any defined group of people, such as a school class, a group of restaurant visitors, or even a country) is called the *primary* case. The people who are infected by this individual are called *secondary* cases. If all of the secondary cases are infected at about the same time, then the *tertiary* cases will also appear approximately simultaneously, and we can talk about waves or *generations* of infection.

Index case

This is the first case to be discovered by the health care system during an outbreak. The finding of this individual leads to an investigation of the outbreak, during which many more cases may be discovered. Often it will be found that there were cases who had fallen ill before the index case was diagnosed.

Thus it is important to note that the index case and the primary case may not be the same person – and in real-life outbreaks they usually are not. However, the terms are frequently used incorrectly.

Reproductive rate

The potential for a contagious disease to spread from person to person in a population is called the *reproductive rate*. It depends not only on the risk of transmission in a contact, but also on how common contacts are – a person with measles who meets no one will not transmit the infection. In a similar way the average rate of acquisition of new sexual partners in a population will influence the spread of sexually transmitted diseases.

The principal determinants of the reproductive rate are as follows:

1. the probability of transmission in a contact between an infected individual and a susceptible one;

2. the frequency of contacts in the population;

3. how long an infected person is infectious;

4. the proportion of the population that is already immune.

Point 2 above is really the most interesting from an epidemiological point of view, and also the most frequently overlooked. The spread of infectious diseases depends not only on the properties of the pathogen or the host, but also in at least equal degree on the contact patterns in the society (who meets whom, how often, and what type of contact they have). We shall examine this further in Chapter 11.

Vector

A vector is an animal, most often an arthropod (e.g. an insect), which picks up the pathogen from an infected person and transmits it to a susceptible individual. The best example is the *Anopheles* mosquito, which is responsible for the spread of malaria.

Transmission routes

Several different classifications exist for the routes of transmission of different infections. These have been generated mostly for the purpose of grouping similar diseases together in handbooks on preventive measures, and none of them is entirely satisfactory. Common classifications include person-to-person spread, air-borne, water-borne, food-borne and vector-borne infections.

An alternative approach would be simply to divide the infections into those that are transmitted directly and indirectly (see Table 2.1).

Most of the infections in the indirect group can also spread through direct contact. In fact, the diseases that are placed in the 'indirect' categories are really just the most infectious ones. If you think about it, there are very few

Table 2.1 Examples of directly and indirectly transmitted infections

Direct transmission	Indirect transmission
Mucous membrane to mucous membrane – *sexually transmitted diseases*	Water – *hepatitis A*
	'Proper' air-borne – *chicken-pox*
Across placenta – *toxoplasmosis*	Food-borne – *salmonella*
Transplants, including blood – *hepatitis B*	Vectors – *malaria*
Skin to skin – *herpes type I*	Objects – *scarlet fever (e.g. on toys in a*
Sneezes, coughs – *influenza*	*nursery)*

infections that could not be transmitted between two people who are as close together as in sexual intercourse. It is only those pathogens that are so weak that they can only spread through this most intimate of contacts that cause what we commonly call sexually transmitted diseases.

The division between sneezes/coughs and 'proper' air-borne spread has been made to highlight the fact that for most air-borne infections one has to be reasonably close to the source, whereas an infection such as chicken-pox can actually spread from one room to the next through the ventilation system.

Of course, there are also infections that do not spread from person to person at all. Most of these are caused by bacteria that live in soil or water, such as those responsible for tetanus and Legionnaires' disease. The epidemiology of such diseases differs very little from that of other illnesses caused by inanimate agents in the environment, such as toxins or radiation.

Reservoir vs. source

A reservoir is an ecological niche where a pathogen lives and multiplies outside humans. For example, freshwater lakes are reservoirs for *Legionella*, voles and other small rodents are probably the reservoir for *Borrelia*, and rodent populations of the Himalayas and Rocky Mountains are reservoirs for *Francisella pestis*.

A source is the actual object, animal or person from which the infection is acquired.

Zoonosis

Zoonoses are infections that can spread from vertebrate animals to humans. Many salmonella infections are zoonoses, as is rabies. Diseases that are spread by insects from person to person, but without a vertebrate reservoir, are not zoonoses.

STI

The term 'venereal disease' is not used much nowadays. For the last couple of decades, the term 'sexually transmitted disease', or STD, has been the correct one. However, since the epidemiology of infections transmitted during sexual intercourse largely concerns asymptomatic infections rather than diseases, the term STD is now being increasingly replaced by 'sexually transmitted infection', or STI, and I shall use this acronym throughout this book.

'Benenson'

Ever since the First World War, the American Public Health Association has published every five years an updated book with guidelines on the epidemiology and control of a large number of infectious diseases. The title of the book is the *Control of Communicable Diseases Manual*, but since its editor during the last quarter of the twentieth century was Abraham S. Benenson, it is usually referred to just as Benenson[2]. This book contains a wealth of information, and is indispensable for anyone involved in the practical application of infectious disease epidemiology. Part of its charm stems from the ordering of diseases in strict alphabetical order, so that 'salmonellosis' is followed by 'scabies' and 'typhus fever' by 'viral warts'.

There are also several definitions of time periods that are important.

Incubation period

The incubation period is not a fixed number of days for any disease, but rather an interval where the middle values are more common than the extremes, and the actual period is often dependent on the infectious dose (a higher dose usually gives a shorter incubation period). The distribution of incubation periods is often skewed to the left, which means that there will be more people with short incubation times than with long ones, and references usually give the median (or mean) period, plus a minimum and maximum.

The incubation period extends from the moment a person is infected until they develop symptoms of disease. During this time they may be infectious, and in fact for many of the common childhood diseases the period of greatest infectivity is towards the end of the incubation period. This fact has important implications for the control of such diseases, since isolation of cases will often occur too late to prevent spread.

Serial interval

For diseases that are spread from person to person, the time period between successive generations is called the *serial interval* (or *generation time*). To be exact, this is the time between the appearance of similar symptoms (e.g. rash, cough) in successive generations. Note that if a person is infectious before they develop symptoms, the serial interval will be shorter than the incubation time.

Infectious period

This is the time period during which a person can transmit a disease.

Latent period

This is the time period from infection until the infectious period starts.

The relationships between all of these time periods are shown in Figure 2.2.

As was pointed out in the previous chapter, a knowledge of these time periods for different diseases is an important diagnostic aid when dealing

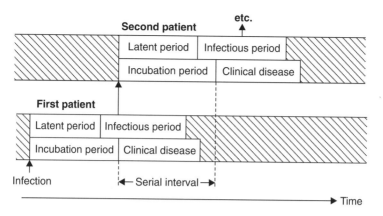

Figure 2.2 The relationships of some important time periods. The patient at the bottom is infected first, and transmits the infection to a second patient.

with individual patients, but it also facilitates tentative diagnoses in outbreak situations. For example, the median incubation time will be much shorter in a calici virus than in a salmonella outbreak. Conversely, if the pathogen that is causing the outbreak is known, knowledge of the incubation time for that disease will make it possible to decide approximately when the exposure must have taken place.

Epidemic

This is one of the most difficult definitions of all, and many suggestions have been made. My favourite, and one of the shortest, is the one in the *Control of Communicable Diseases Manual*, namely 'The occurrence in a community or region of cases of an illness (or an outbreak) with a frequency clearly in excess of normal expectancy'. Some people would probably find this definition too wide, and would prefer to include something about a 'sudden rise in incidence' or 'very large number of cases', while others might want to relate it to the public's perception of this health problem. There is just no universally useful definition.

The word 'epidemic' has an ominous ring to it, and many public health officials prefer to replace it with the more neutral term *outbreak* whenever possible.

When an infectious disease lingers at around the same incidence for a long time, it is called an *endemic*. Many childhood infections may be endemic over a couple of years, only to cause a sudden epidemic every once in a while.

There are also diseases that are endemic in some areas of the world, but which sometimes spread to other places, causing epidemics. The Ganges area is one such endemic area for cholera, a disease that may become epidemic in other places (e.g. Latin America in the early 1990s). In Chapter 11 we shall consider some of the reasons why one disease is endemic and another epidemic.

For the interested reader, the above-mentioned book by John M. Last is a good epidemiological dictionary, and I have tried to adhere to his definitions in this chapter, while adding some personal reflections.

REFERENCES

1. Last JM. *A Dictionary of Epidemiology*, 2nd edn. Oxford: Oxford University Press, 1988.
2. Chin J (ed.). *Control of Communicable Diseases Manual*, 17th edn. Washington, DC: American Public Health Association, 2000.

Chapter 3
Descriptive epidemiology

The first stage of an epidemiological analysis is to present the basic data. This should be done honestly, and the mode of presentation chosen to convey important points clearly to the reader. Some knowledge of what the reader will find interesting is useful.

Descriptive epidemiology never tries to answer the 'why?' question. Its aim is to present existing data on the cases as clearly and comprehensively as possible, using tables, diagrams, graphs or maps. The descriptive work always starts with a list of cases, which is usually entered into a spreadsheet program, or into one of the programs specifically designed for epidemiological analysis. Alternatively, the list of cases may be imported from some pre-existing registry.

The first analysis is done by grouping the cases according to the following:

- time;

- place;

- person.

TIME

In an outbreak, the cases are drawn as an *epidemic curve*. Such a curve has time on the horizontal axis, and the number of cases per time unit on the vertical axis, as shown in Figure 3.1, which depicts an outbreak of salmonellosis in Reykjavik in late summer and early autumn of 2000.

The time unit is usually days, but may be hours in rapid outbreaks (e.g. of gastroenteritis). If the incubation time of the disease causing the outbreak is known, a good rule of thumb is to use one-quarter to one-third of this time as the time unit on the *x*-axis. A good idea, if the outbreak is not too large, is to make one small square for each case, writing the number of each case from the list of cases in the square. This makes it easy to go back and forth between the list and the curve.

The time unit may also be years, as shown in the diagram of annual deaths from variant Creutzfeldt–Jakob's disease in the UK from the first diagnosed cases until 2000 (see Figure 3.2).

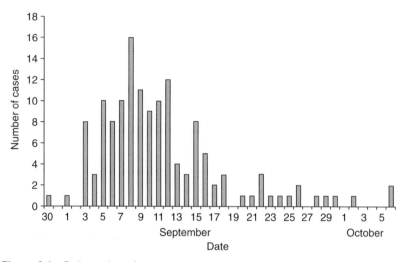

Figure 3.1 Daily number of cases in an outbreak of salmonellosis in Reykjavik in 2000. (Data provided courtesy of Haraldur Briem, State Epidemiologist for Iceland.)

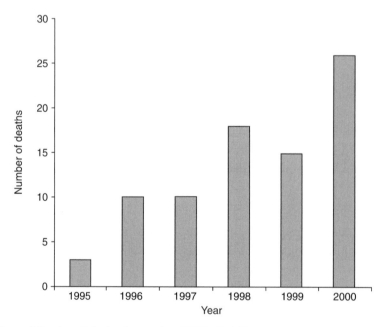

Figure 3.2 Annual deaths from variant CJD in the UK.

In Chapter 12 we shall discuss further how information from an epidemic curve may be used.

Time curves may also be used to describe seasonal variations, such as the incidence peak in late summer and early autumn which is seen in the northern hemisphere for most enteric infections.

PLACE

Geography may of course be described by lists, such as that in Table 3.1, which gives the incidence of some diseases in a number of countries.

This is a straightforward description which immediately raises a number of questions. However, the answers to these are not the task of descriptive epidemiology.

Table 3.1 Reported incidence per 100 000 population in 1999 of some diseases in the countries around the Baltic Sea. (Excerpt from *EpiNorth* 2000; 1: 46–47.)

	Diphtheria	Gonorrhoea	Hepatitis A	Meningococcal meningitis	Salmonella
Denmark	0	6.4	1.7	3.5	61.3
Estonia	0	76.3	26.1	0.4	31.9
Finland	0	4.9	0.9	1.1	54.3
Latvia	3.3	45.1	28.8	1.5	37.5
Lithuania	0.1	30.8	7.2	2.1	39.5
St Petersburg	1.4	128.9	31.8	2.0	41.3
Sweden	0	4.9	1.8	0.6	55.1

Geographical patterns often become more apparent when a map is used, as in Figure 3.3. This map shows the incidence of reported tularaemia cases in Finland during the year 2000, when there was a large outbreak in summer and early autumn.

When drawing a map with different shades or colours for different intervals of the variable shown, one should use not more than five or six levels, or the map will become messy. This may involve some adjusting of the intervals to obtain the right effect, and may also require that the intervals are of unequal length.

If the areas of a map are of widely differing size, and with very different population densities, the map can become quite misleading. A high incidence in a large but sparsely populated region will dominate the impression one gains, even if the dark shading there represents just a few cases. One way to circumvent this problem is to redraw the map with the size of each area (each county in this case) proportional to its population size, but trying to keep the area in its correct position as far as possible, as in Figure 3.4.

This rather odd-looking map gives a much better impression of the absolute size of the outbreak in the various counties.

PERSON

The two standard categories in descriptive epidemiology are sex and age. Since an epidemiologist always wants to break down the data into different categories of age and sex, there is a joke that 'an epidemiologist is someone broken down by sex and age'.

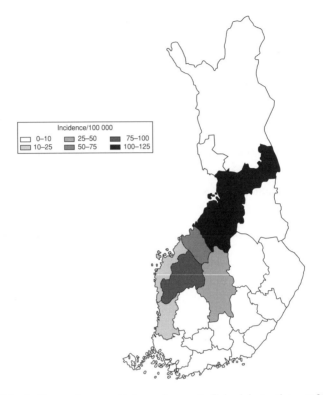

Figure 3.3 Incidence of reported tularaemia cases in Finland during the year 2000, expressed as incidence per 100 000 in the different counties. (Data from Department of Epidemiology, Kansanterveyslaitos; map courtesy of Karin Nygård.)

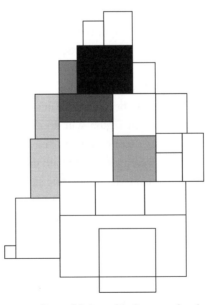

Figure 3.4 Same map as in Figure 3.3, but with the area of each county redrawn so as to be proportional to the number of inhabitants. Shading corresponds to the same incidence values as in Figure 3.3. (Data from Department of Epidemiology, Kansanterveyslaitos; map courtesy of Karin Nygård.)

Sex distribution can be shown in a pie chart, or often more satisfactorily, by just giving the percentages or the ratio of females to males. The well-known population pyramid of demography gives age and sex distribution at the same time (see Figure 12.4 for an example).

Age distribution is usually expressed in intervals, but one of the more irritating failures of the world's population of epidemiologists is our lack of agreement on appropriate age intervals. They are different in almost every publication, which means that you must ask the author for the original data if you want to compare his age distribution with yours. To some extent this failure to agree is due to varying needs in different situations. Paediatricians often want to divide the first year of life into months, or at least have the first category as 0–11 months, the second as 1–4 years, etc. For studies on chlamydia, the common division of age into the groups 10–19 and 20–29 years cuts the age group of most interest, which is usually the 18 to 23-year-olds, into two halves and may dilute interesting findings by including individuals with very different sexual contact patterns in each of the groups.

TABLE OR DIAGRAM?

The choice of whether to display the data as a table or a figure is very much a personal one. To some extent it depends on where and how the descriptive data will be presented. In a lecture, a diagram is almost always preferable, as time will be too short for the audience to study a table, and the main points that one wants to convey will be absorbed much more quickly from a clear graph.

However, in a publication a table is often better. It can contain more exact detail, and if the reader wants to compare your findings with his own, it can be very frustrating to have to use a ruler to try to obtain the exact values of data presented in a graph.

One point should be made about oral presentation. When you show a graph or a table to an audience, always start by saying 'This graph shows. . . .On the horizontal axis we see the . . . and on the vertical axis are the . . .', or 'This is a table of . . . . The columns are the . . . while the . . . are given in the rows', and then pause for a second. After you have given the audience time to orient themselves, you can proceed by pointing to the interesting item in the middle of the picture that you want everyone to observe. Far too often in meetings someone flashes an overhead or computer-generated picture on to the screen and immediately starts pointing to a peak on a curve without giving the audience any chance to understand what this is all about.

The choice between a line graph or a bar graph is to some extent a personal one. Surveillance data over time are often shown as a line, especially if the number of cases is high. Epidemic curves are never drawn as lines, as you can see from several examples in this book. If the variable on the x-axis is categorical (i.e. shows different groups), you should use a bar graph. Do not draw a line between values for a number of ethnic groups, professions, etc.

The most important point to remember when presenting the results of descriptive epidemiology is to be succinct and truthful at the same time – as is of course the case with any statistical analysis. Do not 'improve' your findings by tampering with the axes of a graph, by peculiar grouping of cases, or by selecting just the time interval which proves your point.

A very enjoyable book on how best to present data – and on the many mistakes possible – has been written by E. Tufte[1].

STATISTICAL ANALYSIS

Some simple statistical calculations also form part of descriptive epidemiology. Calculation of averages, standard deviations, percentages, etc., are obvious. Since many of the tests used in the further analysis assume that the data are normally distributed, it is usually a good idea to check this by drawing a graph of the distribution. If it is far from bell-shaped, you might be wise to consult a statistician.

If the subjects studied represent a sample from a larger population, graphs should always have error bars extending up and down from every data point (see Chapter 7 for a longer discussion of samples and confidence intervals). You can choose ±1 standard deviation, ±1 standard error of the mean, or a 95% confidence interval, so long as the text of the figure indicates what they are.

REFERENCES

1. Tufte ER. *The Visual Display of Quantitative Information.* Cheshire, CT: Graphics Press, 1983.

Chapter 4
Risk, relative risk and attack rate

The basic epidemiological concept of comparing risks is introduced, some confusing definitions are discussed, and we meet the attack rate.

A not uncommon situation for a practising physician occurs when several members of a family, a day-care group or a school class fall ill at almost the same time. Often the disease is some type of gastroenteritis, and the patients as well as their doctor wonder whether it might have been caused by something they ate. The answer to that question is complicated by the fact that it is not always possible to single out the meal responsible, and even if one could do so, there are almost always several different food items served during a meal.

AN EPIDEMIOLOGICAL ANALYSIS OF AN OUTBREAK

The situation becomes simpler if a group of people who do not normally eat together share a common meal, and several of them become ill afterwards. The following example shows how one could analyse such a situation by calculating risks and relative risks.

Fifteen people had New Year's dinner together. Within 24 hours, five of them became ill with gastroenteritis. The dinner had consisted of several courses and food items, and the participants had not all eaten the same items. How could the cause of their disease be assessed?

All of the guests were sent a list of the food items that had been served and asked to indicate what they had eaten. As the lists came back, their replies were recorded in a double table, with the guests who had been ill on the left, and the ones who remained well on the right (see Table 4.1).

Table 4.1 Table filled out from questionnaires given to 15 people during an outbreak of gastroenteritis

	Gastroenteritis (5 people)	No gastroenteritis (10 people)
Quiche	||	⊞⊞ |||
Cheesecake	||||	|
Swiss roll	|||	||||
Chocolate cake	|	||
Cheese dip	||||	⊞⊞ ||

The first column tells us that four of the five people who were ill had eaten cheesecake as well as cheese dip. From the second column we can see that only one of the people who did not become ill had eaten cheesecake, but that most people in this group had also eaten cheese dip. Just from looking at this table, we gain the impression that the cheesecake may have been the culprit. How can we check this?

First, we realize that the table is really set up the wrong way. For example, it shows, that if one was ill there was a high probability that one had eaten cheesecake, or that if one remained well there was a strong chance that one had eaten quiche.

What we really want to know is the answer to the opposite question. What was one's chance of being ill if one had eaten cheesecake, or if one had eaten quiche? We therefore rearrange the table (see Table 4.2) in order to ascertain how many guests became ill out of the total who had eaten each item.

Table 4.2 Number of those subjects in Table 4.1 who became ill out of the total number who ate each item

Eaten	Ill	Total
Quiche	2	10
Cheesecake	4	5
Swiss roll	3	7
Chocolate cake	1	3
Cheese dip	4	11

In total, 10 guests ate quiche, and two of these became ill, five ate cheesecake, and four of these became ill, and so on. From these figures we can calculate the risk of becoming ill that is associated with eating each of these food items.

The risk associated with some potentially harmful factor is defined as the proportion who become ill out of all those exposed to the factor.

Two points should be made here about the meaning of the words 'risk' and 'exposed'.

1. Note that epidemiology makes confusing use of the word 'risk'. In everyday language a risk is something that can really cause harm, but in epidemiology it just denotes the statistical likelihood of being ill if one is exposed to some factor – it says nothing about whether this factor really causes the disease. At the beginning of an analysis we do not know which factors (food items in this case) will prove to be harmful, and initially they are all suspects.

2. The use of the word 'exposure' may be even more frustrating, especially for someone with a background in infectious diseases. Normally, when

we say that someone has been 'exposed' to an infectious agent, we mean that they have physically met the bacteria or the virus – someone with influenza has coughed at them, or they have eaten a dish that is known to contain *Salmonella*.

However, epidemiology uses the word 'exposure' to denote having met with a risk factor for the disease, which may or may not be the cause. The difference between the two definitions is sometimes subtle and sometimes confusing. Consider hepatitis B as an example. Known risk factors for acquiring this infection include blood transfusion, intravenous drug use, sexual intercourse, or contact with patients' blood. A person with an acute hepatitis B infection may have been exposed to a number of these risk factors (epidemiological definition), but in only one of these situations were they exposed to the virus (infectious disease definition). The risk factors are only 'causal' if the media involved effectively contain active virus, but they are always 'epidemiological' risk factors, because the media are potential carriers of virus. In another example, someone who has eaten undercooked chicken has been exposed to a risk factor (or has a risk factor) for campylobacter infection, but they may not have been exposed to these bacteria.

(Several modern theoretical epidemiologists also advise against using the term 'risk factor', and propose the much better alternative *determinant,* since this does not imply anything about the cause of the disease. However, this usage is still far from universal, and we shall therefore adhere to common terminology here.)

The word 'factor' is also somewhat loosely defined in this text. This is deliberate – it is used to denote anything that could be associated with risk for disease (a food item, another person, a behaviour, and so on).

To return to the dinner-party example, the risk attached to each food item is calculated as follows:

$$\text{risk} = \frac{\text{number of individuals who ate this food who are ill}}{\text{total number of individuals who ate this food}}$$

i.e. 2/10 for the quiche, 4/5 for the cheesecake, and so on. The risk of illness from eating each of these items is shown in Figure 4.1.

This gives us a list of possibly infected items, with cheesecake and Swiss roll being most suspect, but let us just stop to think for a moment. Suppose that the dinner had nothing to do with the five guests' gastroenteritis, or that the illness was caused by a food item that we forgot to include on the list. The above result may have arisen just by chance.

Now comes the central message of this chapter – we must also look at the risk of being ill among those who did not eat the items on the list. We know that almost half of those who ate Swiss roll were ill, but what conclusion

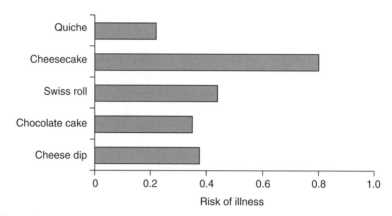

Figure 4.1   Risk of gastroenteritis after having eaten five different food items.

would we draw if we found the same proportion of those who skipped the Swiss roll were ill? The people at the dinner ate many different things, and for most of the items there will be a mixture of those who happened to eat the food and those who did not. If an item was definitely not the cause of illness, we would expect the same risk of being ill whether one ate it or not.

This way of thinking is fundamental to all epidemiology. If an exposure has nothing to do with a disease, then the proportion of individuals who are ill after having had this exposure should be the same as in those who have not had the exposure. We shall return to this way of reasoning several times in this book.

We next proceed to list the outcome according to what people did *not* eat. From Table 4.1, we can see that three of the five guests who became ill did not eat quiche, and that two of the 10 guests who remained well also did not eat quiche, and so on. The full list is given in Table 4.3.

We can then calculate the risk of being ill if one had *not* eaten each of these items, and plot it on a graph together with the risks calculated above (see Figure 4.2).

The figure shows that the risk of being ill is about the same whether or not one ate Swiss roll, chocolate cake or cheese dip. Eating quiche seems almost

Table 4.3   Number of those subjects in Table 4.1 who became ill out of the total number who did *not* eat each item

Not eaten	Ill	Total
Quiche	3	5
Cheesecake	1	10
Swiss roll	2	8
Chocolate cake	4	12
Cheese dip	1	4

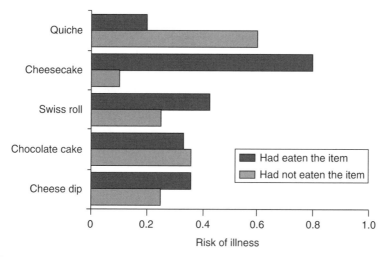

Figure 4.2 Risk of gastroenteritis in those who had and those who had not eaten five different food items.

to have had a protective effect, whereas cheesecake is clearly the most likely culprit, with a risk of being ill of 0.80 in those who ate it, compared with a risk of 0.10 in those who did not.

A simple way of comparing the risks in those exposed vs. those not exposed is to divide them (always putting the risk in those exposed on top). This gives the *relative risk* (also called the *risk ratio*) RR:

$$RR = \frac{\text{risk in individuals exposed to a factor}}{\text{risk in individuals not exposed to that factor}}$$

The relative risks of illness as a result of eating the different food items at the meal are shown in Table 4.4.

Table 4.4 Relative risk (RR) of illness associated with each food item during an outbreak of gastroenteritis

Food	RR
Quiche	0.33
Cheesecake	8.0
Swiss roll	1.72
Chocolate cake	0.93
Cheese dip	1.44

A relative risk of around 1 means that the risk of disease was nearly equal in exposed and unexposed individuals, and that this item is unlikely to have caused disease. A high RR indicates that this item is associated with the disease, and an RR close to 0 would suggest that the item is in some way protective – the risk of disease is then much higher in those not exposed to the item.

From our calculations we find that the RR of causing illness is clearly highest for the cheesecake, and we can conclude with some certainty that this was the item responsible for the gastrointestinal illness.

Two questions remain. First, why was one person ill who had not eaten cheesecake, and secondly, why was one person well who had eaten it? There are several plausible answers to these questions. Perhaps the first person was ill due to something else, or maybe he did eat cheesecake and forgot. Epidemiology is rarely an exact science. The second person could simply have eaten so little of the cheesecake that he did not become ill, since the risk of infection is often related to the dose of the pathogen.

One may also question why the quiche seemed to have a protective effect against illness. One possible explanation is that most guests at the party found it too much to eat quiche *and* cheesecake, so those who ate quiche will be largely the same people as those who did not eat cheesecake, and who thus escaped infection.

PERSON-TO-PERSON SPREAD

The above is an example of infectious disease that is spread from a common source, and we tried to find a likely cause by comparing the relative risks attached to different food items. A quite similar line of reasoning can be applied to diseases that are spread from person to person. In that case we would want to know the risk of acquiring such a disease from an infected person (i.e. how infectious it is).

For most people this is probably the most important issue with regard to communicable diseases, and we all recognize questions such as the following. Can I let my child go to the day-care centre as long as he is infected? What is my risk of contracting meningitis now that my neighbour has got it? What is the risk of HIV transmission during heterosexual intercourse without a condom?

During the years around 1950, Dr Hope Simpson meticulously collected data on all cases of measles, chicken-pox and mumps in a district in western England[1]. One of the issues he wanted to study was the risk of transmission from one child in a family to another. In order to do this he had to register all instances where a child was exposed to a sibling with the disease, and then establish how many of these exposures led to a new case. The results that he obtained during a 4-year period are shown in Table 4.5.

From these figures we can calculate the infectivity of each of these diseases within a family.

The basic measure of infectivity is the *attack rate*.

The attack rate of a disease is the number of cases, divided by the number of susceptibles exposed.

Table 4.5 Numbers of individuals infected out of siblings exposed to three childhood infections (*Source: Hope Simpson*[1].)

	Measles	Chicken-pox	Mumps
Number of children exposed to a sibling with the disease	251	238	218
Number who fell ill	201	172	82

This is really the same as the definition of risk given above. The difference is that here we use the infectious disease definition of exposure, by counting only the individuals who really were exposed to the microbe.

The attack rates will be as follows:

$$\text{measles} \qquad \frac{201}{251} = 0.80$$

$$\text{chicken-pox} \qquad \frac{172}{238} = 0.72$$

$$\text{mumps} \qquad \frac{82}{218} = 0.38$$

Thus four out of every five children exposed to measles in the family will themselves contract measles, and so on. There are clearly appreciable differences in attack rate for these three diseases.

The perceptive reader may note the word 'susceptible' in the above definition of attack rate. How did Hope Simpson know that all of the exposed siblings were still susceptible (i.e. that they had not already had the disease and were immune). The answer is that he did not. He interviewed the parents about previous disease events, but he did not have serology available to ascertain where there had been subclinical infections among the children. This is only a small problem for measles, which is almost never subclinical, but for mumps, which is often quite asymptomatic, he probably overestimated the number of susceptible children. This would lead to a falsely low attack rate for mumps.

In a similar fashion, factors that influence the attack rate can be studied by looking at the number of secondary cases in different groups around a primary case. One obvious such factor is how close one lives to the infected person. In the 1980s there was much concern about the attack rate of monkey-pox, since it was known that vaccination against smallpox also protected against monkey-pox, but as smallpox had been eradicated this vaccination was no longer necessary. In one study, 147 individuals who had caught the monkey-pox virus from monkeys in Zaire were identified[2]. For each case the investigators counted all of the people who had lived in the same residence, and the number of these individuals who became cases. They also tried to calculate the number of more remote contacts that the cases had had, and the number of transmissions to these.

The results were as follows:

Secondary Cases		Healthy	
Same residence	More remote	Same residence	More remote
36	11	798	728

so that the attack rate (= risk) in people who shared their residence with an infective case was:

$$\frac{36}{36 + 798} \text{ (total number exposed in denominator)} = 0.043$$

and in the less close contacts $11/(11 + 728) = 0.015$.

SUMMARY

Whether the number of people who become ill after exposure is high or low does not depend only on the actual number. It must also be compared with the total number who were exposed, and who could have become ill. This is done by calculating the risk.

If we want to find out whether a certain exposure seems to be related to a disease, we must calculate the risk of disease not only in those exposed, but also in those not exposed. The ratio of these two risks tells us the degree of association between the exposure and the illness.

When we are looking at a population where we know that all of the members have been exposed to a pathogen, the risk of acquiring the disease is called the attack rate.

REFERENCES

1. Hope Simpson RE. Infectiousness of communicable diseases in the household (measles, chickenpox and mumps). *Lancet* 1952; **2**: 549–54.
2. Fine PEM, Jezek Z, Grab B, Dixon H. The transmission potential of monkey-pox virus in human populations. *Int J Epidemiol* 1988; **17**: 643–50.

Chapter 5
The case–control study: odds, odds ratios – the concept of confounding

The concept of the case–control study is introduced and odds ratios are defined. We meet the 2 × 2 table and find out whether an odds ratio for a sample can be extended to apply to a larger group. We get acquainted with the subject of confounding, and finally philosophize a little about causes.

In the examples in the previous chapter we had knowledge of the entire population (i.e. we could count precisely how many individuals were exposed and how many were infected). In real life, and especially when studies are based in the community rather than in the clinic, we shall often only have information about some of those who are exposed and some of those who are ill. Such a situation requires slightly different methods. Also in the previous chapter we showed how to assign numerical values for different risks, but we did not discuss how exact and reliable these estimates are. For this we need some statistics.

The first example in this chapter concerns a published outbreak from Wales[1]. In an outbreak of salmonella infection in a large office block where some 1400 people worked, 31 cases were identified among employees and 6 cases among the staff at the canteen. Only three of these 37 cases actually went to a doctor because of symptoms. The rest were found by culturing of faecal samples, or by interviewing for symptoms.

To compare risk factors with people who had not been ill, 58 randomly chosen employees who denied having had any symptoms were given the same questions as the 37 cases. From the dates of first symptoms, and from a knowledge of the incubation period of salmonella infection, it was suspected that the infected food had been served on the 23 January. The questions asked in the investigation were as follows.

1. Did you have lunch in the canteen on 22 January?

2. Did you have lunch in the canteen on 23 January?

3. Did you eat salad on any of these days?

4. Did you eat sandwiches?

5. Did you eat chicken?

The responses to these questions are shown in Table 5.1.

Table 5.1 Results from questionnaires given to 37 cases and 58 controls in an outbreak of gastroenteritis in a large office block (*Source*: Salmon *et al.*[1])

Item	Gastroenteritis		No gastroenteritis	
	Eaten	Not eaten	Eaten	Not eaten
Lunch 22 January	6	31	9	48
Lunch 23 January	18	19	14	43
Salad	12	24	5	52
Sandwiches	16	21	14	44
Chicken	4	33	4	54

In this table we have included the numbers who did not eat each item right from the start, since we know from the previous chapter that we shall need them. In addition, we can see that there must have been some 'don't remember' cases here, because there should have been 37 answers for each item in the group with gastroenteritis, and 58 in the group without the illness.

We would now want to calculate risks and RRs just as in the previous chapter, but that is not possible. If you look back at the definition of risk, you will see that the denominator should include the total number of individuals who had eaten the item. In the New Year's dinner example this was easy, as we were able to interview everyone who had been to the dinner. In the present example we do not know exactly how many people had lunch in the canteen on each of the days, nor do we know how many of them ate the different items on the list. Moreover, it is unlikely that we identified all of the cases. There were probably more employees infected who did not feel ill enough to go to the doctor. Since we know neither the number who were ill nor the number exposed for certain, we cannot calculate any risks.

What we have is an unknown proportion of all of the employees who were ill, and another unknown proportion of all of those who remained well. If the symptoms had been more severe, we would probably have collected a larger proportion of the people who were infected, but we do not know that for certain, and the relative sizes of these proportions are not important for the analysis anyway.

This type of epidemiological analysis is the basic form of a *case–control study*, where risk factors for disease are ascertained by comparing different exposures (in this case the type of food eaten) between individuals who were ill (the cases) and those who were not (the controls). In contrast to the study in the previous chapter, we do not have knowledge of all cases, or of all controls – what we do have are two *samples* of people. Note also that we are doing the analysis 'backwards' in time, starting from a number of cases that were diagnosed, then identifying a number of controls, and after that looking at possible causes of the disease. This retrospective approach is typical of most case–control studies.

The basic idea behind the case–control study is as follows. 'If an exposure is much more common among the cases than among the controls, then this exposure may be associated with the disease – perhaps even a cause.' If some risk factor is only seen in cases, and never in anyone else, then there must be a very strong connection between this risk factor and the development of disease. This is a reverse way of thinking to the analysis in the previous chapter. There we wanted to see whether disease was more common after certain exposures (food items), whereas here we want to find out if certain exposures are more common among the diseased individuals than among the others.

The entity used to measure how common an exposure is, called *odds*, is defined as the number exposed divided by the number not exposed. The analysis begins by calculating the odds connected to each exposure for the cases and for the controls separately.

The odds of having had a certain exposure among the cases is defined as follows:

$$\text{odds for cases} = \frac{\text{number of cases exposed to the factor}}{\text{number of cases not exposed to the factor}}$$

As an example, the odds of having eaten the salad among the cases in the above table would be 12/24 = 0.5; 12 cases had eaten chicken and 24 cases had not. Note that odds are calculated as the ratio of exposed to unexposed, and not as the proportion of all the cases that are exposed. There is a reason for this, to which we shall return in the next chapter.

In a similar way, the odds of having had a certain exposure among the controls is defined as follows:

$$\text{odds for controls} = \frac{\text{number of controls exposed to the factor}}{\text{number of controls not exposed to the factor}}$$

The odds of having been exposed to the salad among the controls is 5/52 = 0.096, and comparing this figure to the odds above, we can immediately see that a higher proportion of the cases than of the controls had eaten salad.

Just as risks could be compared by calculating the relative risk, odds can be compared by a division. The *odds ratio* (OR) associated with a certain exposure is defined as follows:

$$\text{OR} = \frac{\text{odds for cases}}{\text{odds for controls}}$$

which for the salad example would be 0.5/0.096 = 5.21.

The most unfortunate point about odds is that they have less intuitive meaning than the concept of risk. However, even if it is less easy to understand what they really mean, they are readily calculated and extremely useful in the epidemiological analysis.

At this stage we shall introduce the 2×2 (pronounced 'two-by-two') table. It is a cornerstone of all epidemiological research, and often the first thing one draws up when starting to investigate some data.

The general 2×2 table appears as follows:

	Cases	Controls	
Exposed	a	b	a + b
Not exposed	c	d	c + d
	a + c	b + d	Total

where a = number of ill people who were exposed, b = number of well people who were exposed, c = number of ill people who were not exposed, d = number of well people who were not exposed, $a + b$ = total number who were exposed, $c + d$ = total number who were not exposed, $a + c$ = total number of cases and $b + d$ = total number of controls.

(Calling this a 2×2 table is one of the charming inconsistencies of epidemiological terminology – you will notice that this is in fact a 3×3 table. However, the row and column sums do not contain any independent information, and there are thus only two rows and two columns.)

For an infectious disease with very high infectivity, there would not be any individuals in squares b and c. All of the ill people would be exposed $(= a)$, and all of the healthy individuals would be unexposed $(= d)$.

For the factor 'lunch in the canteen on 22 January', our 2×2 table would appear as follows:

	Ill individuals	Well individuals	
Had lunch on 22 January	6	9	15
Did not have lunch on 22 January	31	48	79
	37	57	94

From this table it is easy to calculate the odds and the OR associated with having lunch on 22 January. The odds of having had lunch ('having been exposed to lunch') among the ill individuals is 6/31 = 0.193, and the odds of having had lunch among those who remained well is 9/48 = 0.188. The OR for the risk factor 'lunch in the canteen on 22 January' is 0.193/0.188 = 1.03.

All these odds and odds ratios might seem like an unnecessary complication. Why can we not, as in the previous chapter, calculate the risks from this table (6/15 for the exposed and 31/79 for the unexposed)? The answer is that to do so would be completely wrong! Risks cannot be calculated from these figures, since we know neither the total number who ate or did not eat that day, nor the number of people who were actually infected. We only have our small group of cases and controls, and we can only make statements about them. The calculation of risks and relative risks requires a full knowledge of all of those exposed and of all of the cases.

Similarly, for the factor 'lunch in canteen on 23 January', our 2×2 table would appear as follows:

	Ill individuals	Well individuals	
Had lunch on 23 January	18	14	32
Did not have lunch on 23 January	19	43	62
	37	57	94

Here the odds for exposure are $18/19 = 0.95$ and $14/43 = 0.33$ for the ill and well people, respectively. That is, among the 94 people who answered this question, there was a considerably greater chance of having had lunch on 23 January for those who were infected than for those who were well. The OR for the risk factor 'lunch in canteen on 23 January' is $0.95/0.33 = 2.88$.

In the same way, ORs can be calculated for the three different menu items, and the complete list is given in Table 5.2.

Table 5.2 Odds ratios (OR) for illness associated with each risk factor for the study in Table 5.1

Item	OR
Lunch 22 January	1.03
Lunch 23 January	2.93
Salad	5.20
Sandwiches	2.39
Chicken	1.64

An OR of 1 is equivalent to equal odds for exposure in cases and controls, which is the same as saying that an OR of 1 suggests that this factor is not associated with the disease.

The formula for the odds ratio can be manipulated slightly to give an easier method of calculation:

$$OR = \frac{a/c}{b/d} = \frac{ad}{bc}$$

In other words, multiply the upper left-hand number by the lower right-hand number, and divide by the upper right multiplied by the lower left.

Can we be sure of our ORs?

Our next question is how far from 1 the OR should be for us to regard the factor as being associated with disease. From the above list, we could guess that the lunch on 22 January probably did not contain any infected food items, but how about the lunch on the 23rd? And should the salad be suspected, with its rather high OR? And what about the chicken?

The answer to this question is statistical. We are looking at samples of cases and controls from the total population of 1400 employees. We hope that our sample of cases represents all cases, even the ones that we never found, and that our sample of controls is representative of all those who were not ill, but we cannot be certain of this. It is evident that we could easily just by chance have included a disproportionate number of cases who happened to eat item 'X', or too many of the controls who did not eat item 'Y' compared with their proportion of the total population of controls.

Thus for each of the numbers in the 2 × 2 table there is a statistical uncertainty that affects the exact value of the OR. If we could repeat the same study using other groups of cases and controls, the numbers of answers to each of the questions would probably have been slightly different.

In the ideal world of Plato, a 'true' OR for each of the risk factors does exist, and in principle it would have been attainable by interviewing all of the cases (diagnosing the asymptomatic ones correctly) and all of the controls. By using samples, we are introducing uncertainty, so that if the numbers in squares a or d of the 2 × 2 table happen to be higher than they 'should' have been, then our calculated OR will be too high, and if the numbers in squares b or c are too high, then our OR will be too low. The exact values of our ORs will depend on the sample that we happened to obtain.

The fact that sampling from large populations introduces uncertainty in the numbers calculated is the main reason why statistical methods are so prominent in epidemiology. If you do not understand all of this right now, do not despair, as we shall return to this issue several times in the course of this book.

The probable range of the true OR can be calculated relatively easily from the 2 × 2 table. For each of our five ORs we first calculate something called the *error factor*, which is defined as follows:

$$\text{Error factor} = e^{1.96 \times \sqrt{1/a + 1/b + 1/c + 1/d}}$$

where e is the so-called natural logarithm (= 2.71828...).

This formula might seem complicated, but all of the operations can be performed on a simple calculator. For example, for the exposure 'lunch on 23 January', the calculation would be as follows:

1. First divide 1 by each of the four numbers in the 2 × 2 table, adding the result to the memory of the calculator each time:

$$\frac{1}{18} + \frac{1}{19} + \frac{1}{14} + \frac{1}{43} = 0.203$$

2. Then take the square root of this number: $\sqrt{0.203} = 0.45$.

3. Multiply by $1.96 : 0.45 \times 1.96 = 0.882$.

4. Finally, raise e to this number: $e^{0.882} = 2.41$, which is our error factor.

5. The lower limit of the probable range for the OR for 'lunch on 23 January' is now defined by dividing our calculated OR in the above list by the error factor:

$$\text{lower limit} = \frac{2.88}{2.41} = 1.20$$

6. The upper limit is obtained by multiplying our calculated OR by the error factor:

$$\text{upper limit} = 2.88 \times 2.41 = 6.94$$

The apparently arbitrary number 1.96 that is multiplied by the square root in the formula comes from statistical theory, and is chosen to make sure that there is a 95% probability that the true ('platonic') OR lies between the lower and upper limits, no matter what samples from the larger population chance dealt us. The interval from 1.20 to 6.94 is called a 95% *confidence interval* for this OR. In lay terminology it can be interpreted as follows. 'From the analysis of the sample of cases and the sample of controls that we performed, we can be 95% confident that the true OR for the entire population lies between the two limits.'

You may now wonder why we did not calculate the confidence intervals for the risk ratios in the previous chapter, when we looked at the New Year's dinner example. The answer is quite simple. In that example we had full information for the entire group of people, and the risks and RRs that were calculated applied exactly to that group and to that meal. The figures were what they were, and could not have been otherwise. However, in the present example we sampled from all of the possible people in the office block, and the confidence interval attempts to estimate how much chance in the choice of cases and controls could influence the range of our calculated OR.

In almost all epidemiological studies we look at a sample and try to extend the values found to a larger population. For example, a new antibiotic is tested on a group of patients, and the results are extrapolated to apply to all similar patients. The time from infection with HIV to development of AIDS is measured for a group of patients, and is then extrapolated to apply to all similar HIV-positive individuals. Antibodies to measles are measured in a selected sample of children, and extrapolated to apply to all children in the community of that age. In each of these cases we would not need any confidence intervals *if we only wanted to describe precisely the group we have studied*. However, we usually want our results to be more generally useful, and then each group must be treated as just a sample of a larger population, which means that confidence intervals must be calculated.

A list of the 95% confidence intervals for the five ORs calculated above is given in Table 5.3.

Table 5.3 Ninety-five per cent confidence intervals for the odds ratios (OR) for the study in Table 5.1

Item	OR	95% Confidence interval
Lunch 22 January	1.03	0.33–3.18
Lunch 23 January	2.93	1.21–7.09
Salad	5.20	1.65–16.4
Sandwiches	2.39	0.99–5.80
Chicken	1.64	0.38–7.01

We can see that for each of our risk factors quite a wide range of values are possible for the true OR. The only two confidence intervals that do not include OR = 1 as a possible value are for 'lunch on 23 January' and 'salad'.

This result is formulated as follows. Only for these two risk factors is there statistical evidence that the OR does not differ from 1 merely by chance.

(*Note*: This formula for calculating confidence intervals for an OR is really only valid if all of the four values in the 2 × 2 table are equal to or greater than 10. If any of the values are less than 10, the confidence interval calculated will be too narrow. In Chapter 7, we shall look at how situations with small values in the 2 × 2 table are handled statistically. Also note that the formula requires the actual numbers of the study. They cannot be substituted by percentages of the groups.)

SOME GENERAL POINTS ABOUT CASE–CONTROL STUDIES

In this example, as well as in the New Year's dinner example, we have talked about 'exposures'. This expression should be interpreted in its broadest sense. There are many types of epidemiological studies where the factors we are looking at would not be called 'exposures' in everyday language. For example, if we want to study how condom usage affects the risk of being infected with HIV, then our dividing factor should be whether or not our subjects used a condom. If we want to compare the frequency of infectious mononucleosis in boys and girls, then our dividing variable will be gender. If we want to study whether chicken-pox is a more severe disease in adults than in children, then our dividing variable should be age. Only epidemiologists would call condom usage, gender and age 'exposures', but since you are now studying to be one, you will have to adapt.

The most difficult part of a case–control study is often the choosing of appropriate controls. The cases present themselves, but the controls have somehow to be selected from a suitable population. In the above example we just picked 58 people at random from the list of employees, which intuitively seems like a good choice. If, for example, we had happened to choose employees who never ate at the canteen for controls, our study would have been meaningless. The following definition provides food for thought. A control should be someone who, if he had been infected, would have had the same chance of being included as a case in the study as those individuals who were actually infected. Put the other way around, the controls should be chosen so that, if a case had not been a case, he would have had the same likelihood of being picked as a control as everyone else. Also note from the above example that there is nothing in the theory for case–control studies that prescribes the same number of controls as cases – they could be fewer, or more, or many more.

People who are only vaguely familiar with case–control studies tend to think that each control should be selected to be as similar as possible to his or her corresponding case, except that he or she should not have the disease. However, the proper way to understand the concept is as follows. We have observed that a certain exposure is common among the cases. We now wonder how common this exposure is in the background population of non-cases. In some instances we may know directly that this exposure is generally rare – building on experience and familiarity with the society in which we live. When what was later to be called AIDS was first described as a cluster of *Pneumocystis carinii* pneumonia cases in Los Angeles in 1981, it was noted that the patients were homosexual men. That homosexuality was a risk factor was evident, even without performing any case–control studies since, from experience, it was known that the prevalence of this exposure in the general population would be much lower. (AIDS was in fact initially called 'gay-related immunodeficiency' or GRID.) In a salmonella outbreak in Sweden some years ago, the first eight cases all reported having eaten beansprouts, and we could pin these down as the source, since exposure to fresh beansprouts in the general population of Sweden is not common.

However, two other examples from Sweden highlight the risk of making assumptions about how common an exposure is in the background population. In the first, a Medical Officer of Health interviewed the cases in a small hepatitis A outbreak and learned that almost all of them had eaten ready-made potato salad bought in the stores. His feeling was that buying ready-made potato salad was quite uncommon, and he performed a quick case–control study by just walking into the hall outside his office and asking the first eight people he met if they had eaten this product in the last 3 weeks. To his surprise, seven of them had. In another outbreak of enterohaemor-rhagic *E. coli* (EHEC) in children in a small town, it was found that the majority of the cases had visited a certain hamburger restaurant before falling ill. This seemed to be an important association, but it was soon discovered that a hamburger chain had opened a new restaurant just prior to the outbreak, and that virtually every child in town had been there. This was thus not a rare exposure at all in the background population.

As soon as we have the shadow of a doubt about how common a certain exposure may be in the population from which the cases came, we must perform a proper case–control study.

OTHER EXAMPLES OF CASE–CONTROL STUDIES

Apart from outbreak investigations, as exemplified above, case–control studies have relatively rarely been used in infectious disease epidemiology. One reason for this is probably that the method is of greatest use for the rapid screening of a number of potential risk factors for a disease, which is seldom a problem with infectious diseases. However, there are some noteworthy exceptions. A very nice example comes from an investigation of possible causes of toxic-shock syndrome performed in the USA in 1980[2].

The disease was named in the late 1970s, when it was found that among young adult women in particular there were many cases of a dramatic, rapidly progressing disease caused by *Staphylococcus aureus* toxin, characterized by high fever, compromised circulation and confusion, which sometimes led to death.

At the time of the study, some evidence already pointed to the use of tampons, especially the super-absorbent type, as a risk factor. The investigators telephoned 52 young women who had earlier been diagnosed with toxic-shock syndrome, and asked them if they regularly used tampons during menstruation. Each case was also asked to name a woman friend. The investigators then contacted the 52 friends and asked them the same question. The results were as follows:

	Cases	Friends	
Used tampons regularly	52	44	96
Did not use tampons	0	8	8
	52	52	104

It can be seen that the odds for tampon use in the cases is 52/0 among the cases compared with 44/8 among their friends. Neither the odds for the cases nor the odds ratio can be calculated here, because of the zero in the denominator, but in Chapter 7 we shall learn how to calculate the probability of obtaining this difference in exposure between cases and controls by another method (the probability being less than 0.02 in this study).

Case–control investigations of infectious diseases have, for example, been used to study risk factors for hepatitis C markers[3], and case–control methods have also been suggested for the study of vaccine efficacy[4].

CONFOUNDING

Suppose that a group of people had a meal at which one could choose between fish and meat, and suppose that the mayonnaise that came with the fish was contaminated with bacteria. When one analysed the ensuing outbreak, one would find a high OR for the mayonnaise, but also for the fish, since almost everyone who had eaten mayonnaise had also eaten fish. One could thus be led to believe that the fish caused the outbreak, because of the close association between the risk factor 'mayonnaise' and the risk factor 'fish'. If we had overlooked the fact that mayonnaise was served at the meal, and only compared the exposures 'fish' and 'meat', we would have blamed the fish.

This example illustrates the concept of *confounding*. If we take one group of cases and one group of controls and look for risk factors among the cases, then we may be misled if there is a close association between the real, causative risk factor and some other risk factor.

If we compared the incidence of genital chlamydia infection in skate-boarders with the incidence in people who never skate-board, we would find a higher incidence in the former group, and we might conclude that skate-boarding is a risk factor for chlamydia infection. The *confounding* in this example is due to the fact that on the average the population of skate-board-ers is much younger than the general population, and chlamydia infection is most common among people aged between 18 and 23 years. If we only com-pared cases of chlamydia aged 18 to 23 years with controls in the same age group, the association with skate-boarding would disappear.

Around 1990, the Swedish road safety authorities observed that 5- to 10-year-old small BMWs of the 300 series skidded off the road on curves more often than did other cars. The authorities wanted to recall all of these cars in order to look at their steering mechanisms. An alternative explanation to the finding was that such cars were often bought by young men who wanted a relatively inexpensive but fast car. The factor 'being a young adult male' would be associated with 'driving a not-so-new BMW of the 300 series' and at the same time associated with the outcome 'going too fast round curves'. The apparent relationship between the suspected risk factor 'defective steer-ing mechanism' and 'skidding off the road' would be confounded by the risk factor 'being a young adult male'.

The proper definition is that a *confounder* is a factor which is associated with the exposure one is studying and which is at the same time associated with the outcome. In the fish example, the mayonnaise is the confounder, since it is strongly correlated with the exposure 'eating fish' and at the same time with the outcome gastroenteritis. Strictly speaking, therefore, the confounder need not be the 'real' cause of the disease. It could be any exposure that is associated at the same time with another exposure and with the outcome. In the skate-board example above, age is a confounder even though it is not the cause of chlamydia infection. In everyday epidemiological jargon, the term 'confounder' is loosely used to describe those factors that might influence the strength of the association (i.e. the magnitude of the RR or the OR) between the risk factor we are currently studying and the disease.

When I was a child I was told by my mother not to jump in the piles of fallen leaves that were raked together in the parks in early autumn, because I could contract polio. The observation was statistically true, since that season of the year is strongly associated with the existence of piles of leaves, and it also coincides with the time of maximum transmission of polio virus. However, if one could study leaf-pile jumping at all times of the year, the connection with polio would disappear.

Another good example of confounding comes from a case–control study of risk factors for Kaposi's sarcoma in homosexual men published in 1982, before HIV was discovered[5]. At that time it was speculated that the mutagenic effects of the sexual stimulant amyl nitrite ('poppers') might be responsible for the malignancies observed in these men. Comparing the lifetime usage of amyl nitrite in 20 cases and 40 controls gave an OR of almost 10 for high vs. low frequency of usage, and for several years poppers were discussed as one of the likely causes of AIDS. The confounding comes from the fact that the exposure 'having taken poppers' was closely associated with the exposure 'having had unprotected anal intercourse with many partners', which in turn was closely associated with being seropositive for HIV.

If you read other textbooks on epidemiology, you will find that they devote much more space (often entire chapters) to the subject of confounding. Sometimes this tends to make the problem more complicated than is really necessary. Epidemiology is just as much a question of common sense as of rigid definitions and thorny statistics. If you read that coffee drinkers are at higher risk of pancreatic cancer, you should immediately ask yourself whether there is some other factor that is more common in coffee drinkers than in non-coffee drinkers. Could it be smoking? Or alcohol consumption? The coffee consumption could just be a marker of some more relevant risk factor, and the association due to confounding.

Another example concerns several studies of risk factors for hepatitis B infection in Europeans, which have identified 'injecting drug use', 'blood transfusions' and 'health care work' as being clearly associated with a higher risk of infection, which all seem to be biologically quite plausible. However, they often also cite 'travel abroad' as a risk factor. How does travel in itself give one hepatitis B? The confounding arises as follows. One 'real' risk factor for infection with hepatitis B is unprotected sexual intercourse with someone who is infectious. The prevalence of chronic hepatitis B infection is much higher in many countries outside Europe. The risk factor 'have travelled abroad' will be coupled to the exposure 'have had sexual intercourse with someone who is infectious with hepatitis B', which would be the 'real' risk factor. This is how the confounding occurs.

If data are collected on possible confounders, it is often possible to adjust for confounding in the analysis of data, as we shall see in later chapters. However, this requires that one realizes beforehand what the possible confounders might be, which is again a question of common sense. In the earlier example, if we had forgotten to ask about mayonnaise, we would have believed that the fish was the culprit. An analysis could never adjust for confounders of which it is unaware.

Furthermore, if there is a complete overlap between two exposures – if everyone who had eaten fish had also eaten mayonnaise, and vice versa – it would be impossible to differentiate between these two exposures in the epidemiological analysis. Only if there had been people who had eaten their fish without mayonnaise, or who for some reason chose mayonnaise with meat, would it have been possible to disentangle the exposures.

CAUSATION

The concept of confounding is closely coupled to the concept of *cause*. Have we found the 'real' causative risk factor in our study, or is there a confounder somewhere which we have not observed and which is the real cause of the disease? How can we tell this from an epidemiological study?

The concept of cause is not without its own problems. Consider a situation in which I hit my thumb hard with a hammer while trying to hang a painting on the wall. What causes the pain in my thumb? Is it the hammer, or my clumsiness, or the choice to move to a new home? Is it the improved general economic situation in the country, which made it possible for me to buy a new house? Or is it the inflammatory reaction with oedema and vasoactive peptides in the tissue of my thumb?

This is a silly example, but it highlights the problem of defining precisely the level of explanation at which we want to stop when we are talking about the cause of a disease. Another example concerns the known risk factors for pneumococcal septicaemia, which are as follows:

- smoking;

- alcoholism;

- asplenia;

- old age;

- exposure to a pneumococcus.

If you see a patient with severe pneumococcal pneumonia in the emergency ward, how could you tell which of these risk factors was really the cause of this particular case of disease?

When trying to think about causation it is often helpful to make a distinction between *necessary* and *sufficient* causes. In the above example, exposure to a pneumococcus is a necessary cause – without it there would be no pneumococcal pneumonia. However, it is not sufficient to explain the case, since most people who are exposed to the bacteria will not develop any disease at all. The other four risk factors are neither necessary nor sufficient.

Ingestion of a large number of *Campylobacter jejunii* bacteria is a sufficient cause of gastroenteritis. However, it is not a necessary cause, since the disease 'gastroenteritis' may be caused by a number of other pathogens.

It is only when a disease has a cause that is both necessary and sufficient that we can talk about *the* cause of this disease. There are very few diseases for which such a single cause exists, and that includes the non-infectious ones.

The main pillar of our scientific understanding of the concept of cause is the experiment. If a certain set of conditions always produces the same outcome, then we say that we have discovered the cause of this event. This scientific paradigm – when the same experiment can be repeated by different researchers all over the world and at different times, always giving the same result – lies at the foundation of the remarkable successes in physics, chemistry and other sciences that have been achieved over the last 300 years. From thousands of years of practical experimentation we know that if we throw a stone in the air, it will fall down to the ground, and ever since Newton we have been satisfied with the explanation that gravitation pulls the stone towards Earth. Just as in the above example where I hurt my thumb, there is obviously an explanation at a higher level. What is it that causes this gravitational force? However, in ordinary life this level is not necessary in order to understand and (more importantly) predict the motion of objects in a gravitational field. We are content that we have found a cause when this cause explains and predicts events in the world around us.

Much of the progress in clinical medicine during the twentieth century is also due to experiments, either in the laboratory or in clinical trials involving real patients. In this way, the underlying pathological causes of many diseases and conditions have been revealed. The problem for epidemiology is that it is largely an observational science – we must be content with the 'experiments' that Nature presents to us. We can almost never set up precisely the same set of original conditions and watch the outcome over and over again. Nor can we systematically change the original conditions slightly, one by one, in order to determine how this affects the outcome. Each outbreak, each epidemic, and even each contact between an infectious person and a susceptible one, is unique and will never happen in exactly the same way again.

If it is impossible to perform experiments, how can we make any statements at all about the causes of disease from epidemiological studies? The epidemiological literature is full of discussions of this problem, and the best-known example comes from a paper by the British statistician Sir Austin Bradford Hill in 1965[6]. He lists nine criteria to support the view that an observed risk factor is really the cause of the disease we are observing, but I shall only address three of them, and add some personal comments.

Temporality

This criterion is almost self-evident. In order for a risk factor to be the cause of a disease, it must affect the patient before he or she develops the disease. An example comes from the discussion of the association between infection with *Chlamydia pneumoniae* and coronary heart disease. Genetic material from *C. pneumoniae* has been found in atherosclerotic plaques, but was it there first, or is it just that already existing damage to the endothelium of the vessel wall somehow causes pieces of the bacteria to adhere to it?

Biological gradient

This is one of the strongest criteria for causation. If increasing levels of exposure to a risk factor either raise the incidence or produce more severe disease, then this is strong evidence that we have found a cause. In Chapter 12 we shall describe in some detail the discovery that tick bites transmit Lyme disease, but here I shall merely point out that the relationship between the reported number of tick bites and the risk of disease was one of the early findings that put the researchers on track.

Strength of association

The higher the RR or OR between an exposure and an outcome, the more likely it is that we have found a real cause, since there is usually a limit to the spurious associations that can be caused by confounding. Unfortunately, there is no definition of how high is 'high'. However, values above 100, with nice narrow confidence intervals, should generally make you feel quite satisfied.

One of the other criteria that Bradford Hill lists is 'biologic plausibility'. You should be very careful with this one – there are few observed associations between an exposure and an outcome that could not be given an elegant, highly credible, explanation by a creative research mind. There is still so much within the area of medicine that is unknown or only half known, and so much contradictory knowledge, that most findings could always find some support.

SUMMARY

If we lack information about exposures and outcomes in a clearly defined population, we can conduct a case–control study. Risks cannot be calculated, but instead we use odds and odds ratios, which are based on similar ideas.

Since we are only looking at a sample of all possible cases and controls, there is a statistical uncertainty in the exact figures, which is measured by calculating a confidence interval. We say that a factor is significantly associated with disease if the confidence interval around the OR does not include 1. The most difficult part of a case control study is choosing appropriate controls.

Controls should be selected not to be as similar as possible to the cases, but rather to inform us how common a certain risk factor or exposure is in the background population from which the cases arose.

Even if a factor is significantly associated with disease, this may just be a statistical finding, where the division according to exposure also divides the individuals into high-risk and low-risk groups according to some real risk factor. This is called confounding.

The concept of confounding is closely coupled to the concept of cause, and the observational science of epidemiology will always have a problem with proving that it has found a proper cause of a disease.

REFERENCES

1. Salmon RL, Palmer SR, Ribeiro CD et al. How is the source of food poisoning outbreaks established? The example of three consecutive Salmonella enteritidis PT4 outbreaks linked to eggs. J Epidemiol Community Health 1991; **45**: 266–9.
2. Shands KN, Schmid GP, Dan BB et al. Toxic shock syndrome in menstruating women. N Engl J Med 1980; **303**: 1436–42.
3. Alter MJ, Coleman PJ, Alexander WJ et al. Importance of heterosexual activity in the transmission of hepatitis B and non-A, non-B hepatitis. JAMA 1989; **262**: 1201–5.
4. Smith PG, Rodrigues LC, Fine PEM. Assessment of the protective efficacy of vaccines against common diseases using case–control and cohort studies. Int J Epidemiol 1984; **13**: 87–93.
5. Marmor M, Friedman-Kien A, Laubenstein L et al. Risk factors for Kaposi's sarcoma in homosexual men. Lancet 1982; **1**: 1083–6.
6. Hill AB. The environment and disease: association or causation? Proc R Soc Med 1965; **58**: 295–300.

Chapter 6
The cohort study: rates – the concept of bias

The cohort study is introduced and again we look at risks and risk ratios, now showing how confidence intervals are calculated. We also learn what a person-year is, and how it is connected to rates and rate ratios. We then meet the concept of bias, discuss the merits of a controlled, randomized, double-blind clinical trial, and finally make some comparisons between case–control and cohort studies.

The studies we have been examining in the previous two chapters have all analysed an epidemiological pattern *after* the event has occurred. Sometimes one may be able to plan an epidemiological study a little better in advance. Such studies, in which a defined group of people is followed over time, are probably more familiar to most clinicians than case–control studies.

In a study of HIV infection and tuberculosis in New York[1], 513 intravenous drug users were initially tested for HIV antibody. In total, 215 were HIV-positive and 298 were HIV-negative. They were then followed for any signs of active tuberculosis during an average period of 2 years. The results of the study were as follows:

	Developed TB	No TB	
HIV-seropositive initially	8	207	215
HIV-seronegative initially	0	298	298
	8	505	513

Thus the risk of developing tuberculosis in this group was $8/215 = 0.037$ for those who were seropositive at entry, and $0/298 = 0$ for those who were seronegative.

This type of study, in which one first defines and measures the risk factor that one wants to evaluate (in this case HIV status) in a defined group, and then follows this group over time to see who develops the outcome (in this case TB), is called a *cohort study*.

Note the use of the word 'outcome' in the above paragraph. It is quite a useful term when discussing epidemiological theory. In most instances the outcome we are studying is a disease, but it could well be other things, such as the absence of disease after an intervention programme, or a behaviour change after some type of educational campaign. As epidemiology has evolved increasingly into a scientific branch of its own, the more specific terms 'risk factor' and 'disease' are increasingly exchanged for the more general terms 'determinant' (or 'event') and 'outcome'.

As another example of a cohort study, there has been much discussion about whether sexually transmitted diseases, and especially genital ulcerative disease, increase the risk of HIV transmission. In a study from Nairobi[2], Cameron et al. followed 293 men who presented at an STD clinic. They all reported having had sexual intercourse with women from a group of prostitutes among whom HIV infection was known to be common. About half of the men presented with an ulcerative disease, and the rest presented with urethritis. After the first visit, the men were tested repeatedly for 3 months to see if they had also seroconverted in an HIV antibody test (which may take several weeks to become positive after the actual transmission). The results were as follows:

	Seroconverted	Remained HIV-negative	
Presented with genital ulcers	21	128	149
Presented with another condition	3	141	144
	24	269	293

The RR of seroconversion for the factor 'ulcerative disease' was thus 21/149 divided by 3/144 = 6.8.

The authors concluded that the men who were infected with ulcerative disease were infected with HIV in the same intercourse, and that women who had an ulcerative disease were also more likely to transmit the HIV virus.

In contrast to the case–control study in the previous chapter, where risks and relative risks could not be calculated, we can always use risks and RRs for our comparisons in a cohort study, since we have started by defining the total group of people that we want to study.

In a similar manner to the ORs of the previous chapter, we need some way of determining the precision of our calculated RRs. We need to know how much the 'true' RR could differ from the one that we have found, and specifically if it is possible that the RR could be 1 (which would mean that we cannot deduce that the factor we are analysing is associated with disease).

The way to calculate a confidence interval for an RR is almost the same as for an OR. We first calculate the error factor for a relative risk:

$$\text{error factor} = e^{1.96 \times \sqrt{(1/a + 1/b)}}$$

and then divide and multiply the RR with this value to obtain the lower and upper limits, respectively, just as for odds ratios in the previous chapter. (You may wonder why the last two terms under the root sign are 'missing' here, compared with the error factor for the OR. Put simply, this is because in a cohort study the exact number of people in both groups is fixed from the start, and therefore there is no chance variation in these numbers, as there was for c and d in the case–control study.)

For the RR of the Nairobi study, a very approximate calculation would be as follows:

$$\text{Error factor} = e^{1.96 \times \sqrt{(1/a + 1/b)}} = e^{1.96 \times \sqrt{(1/21 + 1/3)}} = e^{1.96 \times 0.62} = 3.37$$

and the lower and upper limits for our confidence interval would be $6.8/3.37 = 2.02$ and $6.8 \times 3.37 = 22.9$, respectively. Thus the confidence interval seems to be well above $RR = 1$, but since the above formula requires that both a and b are at least 10, this approximate interval cannot be trusted completely.

A cohort study does not have to be *prospective* (i.e. a study in which the subjects are entered at that time and subsequently followed into the future). If there is a way of collecting a cohort that was defined at some time in the past, it is possible to save a lot of time by looking at its members now. This is usually called a *retrospective* cohort study.

There has been some debate about whether acute infectious myocarditis predisposes to chronic cardiomyopathy with heart failure later in life. In a study undertaken in 1986[3], 44 of the 45 patients who had been hospitalized at one hospital in Stockholm for acute myocarditis in 1968 and 1969 were contacted. They had then been part of a study to ascertain the microbiological aetiology of their condition, and had been diagnosed and investigated rigorously. Just by sending them a questionnaire it was possible to show that their risk of having any heart disease did not differ from that of the average population. In this way, a 17-year follow-up was achieved within a few months.

This study used the average population as the non-exposed group, which is quite common in cohort studies. In doing so, one implicitly assumes that the proportion of individuals exposed to the risk factor in the average population is low. Ideally, the control group should only consist of people who had never been exposed to the risk factor (i.e. who had never had myocarditis in this case), but this condition is difficult to fulfil when one is using published national health statistics for the comparison. However, if the disease is rare, the influence of the few exposed individuals on the overall frequency of the disease in the overall population will be greatly diluted.

PERSON-YEARS

One problem in the analysis of cohort studies is that all subjects are rarely observed for the same time period. They may enter the study at different times and they may be lost to follow-up at different times. In a large study over a long time period, it is inevitable that the investigators will lose contact with some of the individuals.

The way to deal with this is not to use the number of people in the exposed and unexposed groups for the calculation of risks, but rather the sum of times each person has been followed up. Therefore for each individual in the study one measures the time from entry either until that person becomes ill, or until they are lost to follow-up, or until the study is terminated. This time becomes the observation period for each person, and these times are added for all individuals in each group. Most often the numbers of months or years are added, and the number of people who become ill is divided by the number of person-months or person-years experienced by all of the subjects in the group. Figure 6.1 illustrates this principle.

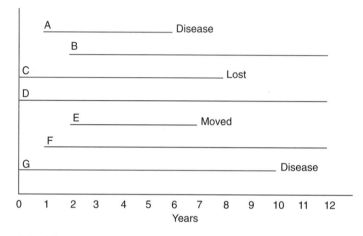

Figure 6.1 Schematic representation of a cohort study. Each line from A to G represents the monitoring period for a patient.

Seven people who are at risk for some disease are followed in a cohort study that lasts 12 years. Subject A enters the study after 1 year, and becomes ill after 6 years. He contributes 5 person-years. Subject B enters after 2 years, and is still well at the end of the study, thus adding 10 person-years. Subject C is followed from the start, but the investigators lose contact with him after 8 years, and so on. The total number of person-years in this study would be 5 + 10 + 8 +12 + 5 + 11 + 10 = 61.

RISKS AND RATES

One of the most abused terms in epidemiology is the word *rate*. This word should mean something that has to do with changes over time (i.e. how quickly something is happening). However, it is very often taken to mean just 'proportion' or 'percentage'. This practice is confusing to the novice entering the field of epidemiology, and should be discouraged. It should be realized, though, that for some concepts, such a change in terminology will probably be a long time in coming. A good example is the term 'attack rate' which we met in Chapters 2 and 4. This is not a rate at all, but rather a proportion or a percentage. (For a most enjoyable discussion of the words rate, ratio and proportion, see reference 4.)

Here, we need to use the term *rate* in its proper sense to describe the situation in Figure 6.1, because if we look back to the definition of risk in Chapter 4, it is 'the proportion who become ill out of all those exposed to a factor'. This definition is clear for an outbreak, when everyone who became ill did so within 24 hours, but what happens if we follow outcomes to exposures over much longer periods? The long-term risk of dying after exposure to any risk factor is always 100%, because as the author says, 'in the long run we are all dead'. The risk of becoming infected with a pathogen that exists around us, such as herpes, TB or campylobacter, is evidently greater the longer the time interval one considers. In short, the figure for a risk depends on the time period.

This problem does not adhere to the concept of a rate, and it is defined as follows:

*The **rate** is the number of subjects who fall ill, divided by the total time under study added by all of the subjects in the cohort.*

In Figure 6.1, there are two individuals who acquire the disease during the 61 person-years of the study. The rate is calculated as the number who become ill divided by the total number of person-years, or in this case 2/61 = 0.033 per person-year. In using a rate, we assume that all person-years are comparable, so that there will be the same number of cases whether we follow 100 subjects during 1 year or 10 subjects for 10 years (the predicted number of cases in this example being 3.3 for both studies).

If the subjects in Figure 6.1 were patients who were hepatitis B surface-antigen (HBs Ag)-positive and the disease was cirrhosis, we could compare them with another group of individuals who were HBs Ag-negative, and then calculate the rate of development of disease in that group. Just as for RR and OR, we could then divide them to yield a rate ratio, which would show by how much HBs Ag positivity increased the rate of contracting cirrhosis.

The confidence interval for a rate ratio is calculated just as for an RR – that is, by first obtaining the error factor

$$EF = e^{1.96 \times \sqrt{(1/a + 1/b)}}$$

where a is the number of people who fall ill in the first group, and b is the number in the second group (both should be greater than 10 for the formula to apply properly). The rate ratio is then divided by the EF to obtain the lower limit, and multiplied with it to obtain the upper limit.

BIAS

Bias is probably a much more familiar concept to most clinicians than confounding. It is concerned with the representativity of our subjects and our data. Are the patients in the study really a good sample of all of the patients we want to make inferences about? Is the same attention given to the subjects in the case group and the control group? Do the subjects in both groups respond to our questions with equal honesty?

The ability to discover possible biases requires a combination of common sense and clinical experience. Some examples are listed below.

1. It would obviously be misleading to use the patients with salmonella in an infectious disease ward for a study of the clinical symptoms and complication risks of a salmonella infection. These patients would be much more seriously ill than the average salmonella infection case (since they were referred to a hospital).

2. The proportion of people infected with HIV in a country can hardly be estimated by the percentage of HIV-positive blood donors. Since people who may be suspected of being at high risk of HIV infection are actively discouraged from donating blood, this figure must surely be an underestimate.

3. People who are given a new vaccine will be closely scrutinized for adverse reactions. If we do not follow a comparison group that should ideally be injected with another, previously well-studied vaccine or some inert substance just as closely, we are likely to overestimate the risk of mild adverse reactions in the group given the new treatment (since many mild reactions, such as headache or general malaise may have nothing to do with the vaccine, and should be just as common in the control group).

4. In a case–control study of an outbreak, the cases are probably more likely to remember exactly what they ate, since they will already have suspected the meal, and they may have thought through or talked through the different possible dishes that could have been responsible.

Examples 1 and 2 represent *selection biases,* example 3 represents an *observer bias,* and example 4 represents a *response bias.* When you design a study, or read one that has been published, you should use your experience and carefully consider the different biases possible.

Another bias may be introduced by so-called *losses to follow-up.* Every cohort study has the problem that not all of the subjects can be followed until the end of the study. As indicated in Figure 6.1, some people move, some die from something other than the disease we are studying, and some just lose contact. If subjects are lost at random, this is not a major problem, and it will only mean that there will be lower numbers on which to base the calculation of RRs, and the confidence intervals will be wider. However, if there is some association between the probability of being lost and the outcome (e.g. that the people who remain healthy cannot be bothered to come back to the clinic to be examined again), then our study will be seriously affected.

In such instances, one usually makes some attempt to contact all of the losses to follow-up, and a few more will be brought into the fold. However, some subjects will still not come, and we shall continue to wonder whether we have a bias. It might often be a better use of resources instead to draw a smaller (10% or so) random sample of all of the losses to follow-up, and really put all one's efforts into obtaining the data for them.

CLINICAL TRIALS

A clinical trial is really a special example of a cohort study. As was pointed out in the previous chapter, the major conceptual difference between an epidemiological study and a clinical trial is that in epidemiology we generally cannot control the risk factors or exposures of the subjects – we have to be satisfied with the way in which nature or chance has set up the 'experiment' for us. In clinical trials, on the other hand, we can choose the subjects at will, and also assign different exposures (most often types of treatment) to different groups.

The golden standard of all such research is the *placebo-controlled, randomized, double-blind* clinical trial. Reflecting on the merits of this research strategy is good practice for thinking about confounding and bias. Let us look at each of these three terms in turn.

Placebo-controlled trials

When we subject a group of patients to a new treatment, we can usually observe changes. The patients may be feeling better, they may have lower values for their liver enzymes, or they may be able to leave hospital earlier. The problem is that we often cannot be sure that these improvements are not caused by chance, or by something else that has changed since we started the treatment. If the improvement is really due to some other concurrent change in treatment, we would have a good example of confounding. The difference in outcome that we ascribe to our new treatment would really be explained by some associated event.

The way to solve this problem is to have a *control* group of patients with the same disease, who receive exactly the same treatment as the study patients, except for the factor that we want to study. Ideally they should be given some inactive treatment (which is called a *placebo)*, or the previously best available treatment. The situation is rather like the comparison of risk of gastroenteritis from eating cheesecake described in Chapter 4, where the group who did not eat cheesecake supplied a measure of risk of disease in the control group. In any clinical trial, the changes in the group on active treatment should be compared with the control group to see whether the differences indicate a real effect.

Several studies have shown a so-called 'placebo effect' of around 30% in clinical trials, which means that around 30% of patients will experience some effect even from totally inactive substances. Probable explanations for this are simply people's expectations, or the increased attention they receive from their doctor when they are the subjects of some type of trial.

Randomized trials

When we have a group of patients and want to assign them to two (or more) different treatments, a number of biases are possible. If we let the patient choose the treatment, it is conceivable that certain types of patients will choose certain options, which could mean that the groups do not become similar with respect to other important variables. If the physician makes the choice, he might allocate patients to the different groups according to his pre-conceptions of the new treatment (if he believes strongly in the new therapy, there may be a tendency to allocate the really ill patients to the treatment group, but if he is uncertain about its merits, it may be the other way around).

Randomization ensures that there is no bias with regard to which patient receives which treatment. If the groups are large enough, it also tends just by chance to make the two groups similar in all variables that may cause confounding, such as age, sex, etc. For small groups this may not be the case, and in the analysis one should always check that the groups are comparable with regard to possible confounders (same average age, equal proportion of men and women, etc.).

Double-blind trials

The word 'blinding' implies being ignorant of whether or not the patient is taking the active drug. 'Single-blind' means that the patient does not know, but the physician does. In a 'double-blind' trial, neither of them knows. There are even 'triple-blind' trials, where the statistician evaluating the outcome of the study is also kept ignorant of the meaning of the group assignments until after the analysis is completed.

Blinding may be important, since even if there is a good control group and treatment has been randomized, it is still possible that the patient's or the physician's preconceptions about the new therapy will influence the results. This is particularly a problem when the outcome variables are more or less subjective as, for example, with insomnia or headache, but even if the variables measured are 'hard figures', physician knowledge of the allocation group may still influence the frequency of blood tests or interpretation of borderline values.

By ensuring that both the physician and the patient are blind to which group the patient belongs to, such biases can be eliminated. Double blinding is of course only possible if there is an alternative therapy that cannot be distinguished from the one under trial (i.e. almost exclusively in tests of drugs). A study of surgery vs. antibiotic therapy in the treatment of brain abscess can hardly be blinded. Even in placebo-controlled tests of drugs it may often be possible for the physician to guess whether the patient is on active treatment or not from the results of blood chemistry.

PROS AND CONS OF CASE–CONTROL AND COHORT STUDIES

This and the previous chapters have introduced the concepts of case–control and cohort studies. It may not be entirely clear why sometimes one is chosen for an epidemiological study and sometimes the other.

One important conceptual difference between the two types of study is concerned with time. In a cohort study we start with a number of subjects who are free from disease, and follow them over time to see who becomes a case and who does not. In a case–control study, the events have already happened before the study started, and we collect the cases and try to find appropriate, disease-free controls.

This means that in many instances the choice of method is actually governed by the available data. Cohort studies usually require carefully planned, often lengthy investigations, whereas a case–control study can quite often be performed quickly from a number of cases that have already been collected.

Another important deciding factor concerns the incidence of the disease that one wishes to study. For diseases with a very low incidence, cohort studies may not be practical or even feasible. Suppose we had a suspicion that the use of dental floss is a strong risk factor for developing infectious endocarditis. The repeated small traumas to the gums caused by pulling these plastic bands back and forth between the teeth could serve as portals of entry into the bloodstream for the alpha streptococci of the mouth. Endocarditis is a very rare disease, and it seems quite clear that most people who use dental floss do not develop it. If we wanted to study this question in a cohort fashion, we would probably need to collect one huge group of dental floss users and one of non-users, and then follow them for a long time to see whether any cases of endocarditis appeared. It is doubtful whether such a study would be feasible. In the case–control mode, we would instead approach a number of people who had already been diagnosed with endocarditis and ask them if they were dental floss users. We would then calculate the proportion of 'yes' answers in this group and compare the result with the proportion of users in a similar group of people who had not had endocarditis, and so obtain an odds ratio for usage in the group of cases. The latter approach would obviously be very much faster and cheaper.

On the other hand, if the incidence of the disease is high, it might be just as easy to collect a cohort and follow them as to get involved in the delicate business of finding adequate controls. This is especially true as problems with bias and confounding are often worse in a case–control than in a cohort study. If we wanted to study the efficacy of an influenza vaccine during an epidemic season, the simplest approach would probably be to randomly vaccinate half of a defined group of subjects and follow the entire group for a couple of months. A case–control study in this situation would involve comparing vaccination status in cases and non-cases of influenza, and it could be difficult to make certain, for example, that there were no confounding factors with regard to who had been vaccinated and who had not.

Another primary conceptual difference concerns the measures of strength of association in the two types of studies – the ORs and the RRs. As was pointed out in Chapter 5, an odds ratio does not have any directly interpretable meaning. It just tells us how strongly an exposure and an outcome seem to be related to each other. In the dental floss example above, a case–control study might reveal a very strong and statistically significant relationship between floss usage and endocarditis. However, this OR would not tell us what we really want to know, namely what is the risk of developing endocarditis if one uses dental floss regularly for, say, 30 years. To answer this question, we need a study that could measure the risks, and we are left with the option of an impossible cohort study.

However, theoretical developments in epidemiology during the last few decades have shown that in some instances the OR obtained from a well-performed case–control study could serve as a good approximation to the usually more relevant RR. This is especially true if the disease is rare both in those who have the risk factor and in those who do not, as can be shown by looking at the general 2×2 table again:

	Ill subjects	Healthy subjects	
Exposed subjects	a	b	$a + b$
Not exposed subjects	c	d	$c + d$
	$a + c$	$b + d$	

If this had been the result of a regular cohort study, we would have said that the risk of disease in the exposed subjects was $a/(a + b)$ and that in the non-exposed subjects was $c/(c + d)$. The relative risk of becoming ill for someone who was exposed would be

$$RR = \frac{a/(a + b)}{c/(c + d)} = \frac{a(c + d)}{c(a + b)}.$$

However, if this was a rare disease, this means that in the total population the number of unexposed ill people (c) would be very small compared with the large number of unexposed healthy people (d). The sum ($c + d$) would thus be almost the same as d only. Similarly, the number of exposed people who became ill (a) would be very small compared with all of the people who were exposed but remained healthy (b), and thus ($a + b$) $\approx b$.

The relative risk of disease would accordingly be as follows:

$$RR = \frac{a(c + d)}{c(a + b)} \approx \frac{ad}{cb}$$

which happens to be the definition of the odds ratio!

Here lies an interesting twist in the way to look at case–control studies and odds ratios. You will remember from Chapter 5 that the idea behind case–control studies is to find out whether some exposure is more common in cases than in controls, but as was pointed out in the example with dental floss, the interesting question is not what sick people were exposed to, but rather how dangerous the exposure is to healthy people. In the discussion of ORs in the previous chapter, I also emphasized that odds are calculated as the number of exposed individuals divided by the number of unexposed subjects, not as the number of exposed individuals divided by the whole group (of cases or controls). This way of defining odds, together with the rules of mathematics, thus leads to the finding that for rare diseases an OR often provides a good approximation to the RR.

In fact, it can be shown that depending on how the controls are chosen, we can obtain an OR that is an estimate either of the classical odds ratio, or of the relative risk, or of the rate ratio even for diseases that are not rare[5]. I shall not go into the details of those theoretical discussions here, but merely point out that the times at which the controls are chosen are important.

In a 'classical' case–control study, one collects a set of cases and then looks around for disease-free controls. Hopefully these will be selected in a way that avoids biases, and data on possible confounders should be recorded. Another approach would be to identify a control for each case just at the time when the case falls ill. This means that a person who was originally chosen as a control could well become a case later, but that does not disqualify them from remaining as a control in the study. It can be shown that an OR calculated from such a study becomes a good approximation of the rate ratio of disease between exposed and non-exposed subjects.

One note of caution should be given concerning the use of case–control studies to estimate relative risks and rates. Even if the methods suggested seem attractive and have good theoretical foundations, they still always assume a completely unbiased choice of controls. Probably the most important condition is that the selection of cases and controls should not be based on exposure status or, stated even more formally, the exposure distribution in the controls should be an unbiased estimate of the exposure distribution in the population from which the cases were drawn. When reading the results of any case–control study, one should always ask the following questions. How were the cases selected? How were the controls selected? Could there be any systematic difference between the two selections, so that the groups are not really representative of the same population?

The final deciding factor when choosing the type of study to use is not infrequently cost. There is a well-known joke among epidemiologists that 'No researcher will ever be able to undertake a cohort study, since when one is old and well recognized enough to get the large funds necessary, one will be too close to retirement to be able to follow the project through to completion, and when one is young enough to have time to see the project through to its completion, one will be too unproven to attract the kind of research money that is needed.'

SUMMARY

In cohort studies we follow defined groups of people over time to see how many of them develop disease. By dividing this figure by the original number of subjects, we can calculate the actual risk of disease in each group. In real life, the subjects of a cohort study often enter it at different times, and it becomes practical to use the total time in the study (i.e. person-years or person-months) to calculate what proportion fall ill per person-time unit, which is then called the rate.

Cohort studies often take a long time, and it is important that all of the participants are followed up for the entire study, or at least that the causes of loss to follow-up are known for each subject. If we selectively lose contact more with one group of subjects than with the other (e.g. if the people we denote as 'losses to follow-up' have in reality died from the disease we are studying), then our estimate of risk or rate will be biased.

Bias may be introduced either by the selection of subjects or by the way in which data is collected. Avoidance of bias requires careful consideration when a study is planned, as once it has been introduced, it may be impossible to adjust for it in the analysis of the data.

A controlled, randomized, double-blind trial tries to eradicate confounders (known and unknown) and biases by letting chance determine who is allocated to which group, and by precluding patient and observer bias. If confounding variables are to be equally distributed between the groups, these cannot be too small, since chance may easily play tricks with small numbers.

The choice between performing a cohort study or a case–control study is often governed by considerations of time and money. In general, cohort studies have fewer problems with bias, but are more time-consuming and expensive.

REFERENCES

1. Selwyn PA, Hartel D, Lewis VA et al. Prospective study of tuberculosis among intravenous drug users with human immunodeficiency virus infection. N Engl J Med 1989; **320**: 545–50.

2. Cameron DW, Simonsen JN, Lourdes JD et al. Female-to-male transmission of

human immunodeficiency virus type 1: risk factors for seroconversion in men. *Lancet* 1989; **2**: 403–7.

3. Giesecke J. The long-term prognosis in acute myocarditis. *Eur Heart J* 1987; **8**: 251–3.

4. Elandt-Johnson RC. Definition of rates: some remarks on their use and misuse. *Am J Epidemiol* 1975; **102**: 267–71.

5. Rodrigues L, Kirkwood B. Case–control designs in the study of common diseases: updates on the demise of the rare disease assumption and the choice of sampling scheme for controls. *Int J Epidemiol* 1990; **19**: 205–13.

Chapter 7
Some statistical procedures that are often used in epidemiology

Here we take a practically oriented look at some of the simple statistical methods and procedures that may be useful for preliminary analysis of data. The confidence interval for a proportion is described, and the t-test is introduced. The χ^2 test is presented at some length, and Fisher's test gets a mention. Finally, some common misconceptions about significance testing are discussed.

This is not a statistics textbook, and a large number of very good medical statistics books have been published. However, there are a number of simple statistical calculations that are often very useful in epidemiology, most of which can be performed on a pocket calculator. It gives one a certain feeling of self-confidence to be able to provide an approximate confidence interval for data one has produced, or to be able to check the calculations in a published paper one is reading. This chapter includes some statistical procedures that I myself have often found useful, including a few round estimates that can even be done in one's head.

Two procedures have already been introduced in the previous chapters, namely how to calculate 95% confidence intervals for odds ratios and for relative risks. This can be done quickly, and gives a sense of the possible ranges of the ORs and RRs, although you will find that for a surprising number of real studies the requirement that all cells of the 2×2 table must have a value of 10 or greater does not hold.

Another procedure that is not uncommon in epidemiology is to estimate the confidence interval for a proportion.

CONFIDENCE INTERVALS FOR PROPORTIONS

Often one wants to estimate the proportion of the population that have some characteristic, such as the proportion who have antibodies to disease A, or the proportion of the population who have had a test for disease B. It is seldom possible to test or ask every member of the population, so one would probably do this by collecting a random sample.

The fundamental assumption in the calculations below is that this sample is truly random, with no selection biases involved. That is, every member of the population we want to describe should have the same chance of ending up in our sample. Our question would be how the proportion measured in the sample relates to the true prevalence in the population. This is exactly the same reasoning that we followed in Chapter 5 with regard to the confidence interval for ORs. If one only wants to make a statement about the sample just studied, there is no need for confidence intervals. If 31 out of 100 subjects tested have antibodies to hepatitis A, then the seroprevalence in this group is 31%, and could not be otherwise. However, this is a very rare situation, and one usually wants the results to be applicable to some larger population.

One intuitively feels that the size of the sample is important. If three individuals out of a sample of ten had antibodies to hepatitis A, then chance could play a major role. The 'true' seroprevalence in the population could easily have been closer to 20% or 40%, and one would hesitate to state that it was 30%. However, if we took a sample of 100 subjects out of a large population and found 31 individuals to be seropositive, we would feel more certain about the estimate of 'about 30%', and even more so if 308 out of 1000 subjects sampled were found to have antibodies. The larger the sample, the less influence there will be from the random inclusion of a couple of seropositives 'too many' or 'too few'.

The confidence interval for a proportion is calculated in the following manner.

1. Write the number as a proportion instead of as a percentage. For the last sample in the above paragraph the proportion would be 0.308 (308 out of 1000 individuals tested).

2. Call this proportion p (note that this is not at all the same p as when we talk about probabilities and statistical P-values, it just uses the same abbreviation.) Call the total number of subjects in the study n.

3. Calculate the number $p \times (1 - p)/n$. In our example this would be $0.308 \times 0.692/1000$.

4. Immediately take the square root of this number

$$\sqrt{(p \times (1 - p)/n)} \text{ or in the example } \sqrt{(0.308 \times 0.692/1000)} = 0.015.$$

5. This number is called the *standard error of a proportion*.

6. Just as we obtained the error factor in the previous chapters, we now multiply the standard error by 1.96, and again this is a statistical device to create a 95% confidence interval:

$$1.96 \times 0.015 = 0.029$$

7. However, this time we do not divide and multiply by our final number, but instead we subtract and add it to the original proportion (0.308 in the example):

Lower limit: $0.308 - 0.029 = 0.279$
Upper limit: $0.308 + 0.029 = 0.337$.

8. In words, we assume that we have taken a truly random sample (no biases) of 1000 subjects out of a much larger population. In this sample we have found 308 subjects to be positive for hepatitis A antibody. We can then state that with 95% probability the true seroprevalence in the population must be between 27.9% and 33.7%.

Note the caveat about bias. If the sample was biased in some way, the calculated proportion will be false and the confidence interval will be meaningless. If we asked 1000 people if they had had an HIV test, but several of those who had had a test said that they had not, then our calculated proportion for the total population would be too low, and this problem is in no way solved by adding a confidence interval to the figure. The confidence interval only shows the possible influence of chance (or *sampling error*) – it cannot be expected to read people's minds.

An approximate estimate

As you can see from the formula, the width of the confidence interval for a proportion is approximately equal to the square root of n. The interval is widest when the proportion is around 50%, and narrows when it gets closer to 0 or to 100%. A quick estimate of how many percentage units up or down the interval would reach is given by the following:

$$CI \approx \pm \frac{100}{\sqrt{(n)}}\%.$$

Therefore if we find a value of 40% for a proportion in 10 subjects investigated, the approximate 95% confidence interval would range from $40 - 30 = 10\%$ up to $40 + 30 = 70\%$. For 100 subjects, the 'true' value in the background population could be 10 percentage units up or down, and with 1000 subjects it would be around ± 3 percentage units.

If we compare two samples of, say, 100 subjects, the difference must accordingly be rather large to be statistically significant. Let us assume that we wanted to see how the proportion of methicillin-resistant *staphylococcus aureus* (MRSA) in different hospitals was related to a particular hygiene practice. If we took 100 samples from patients in each hospital, and found one of them to contain 20% MRSA, the proportion of MRSA in the next hospital would have to be almost 40% for the difference to be statistically significant (i.e. the respective 95% confidence intervals should not overlap).

THE CONFIDENCE INTERVAL OF ZERO

A not uncommon event in epidemiology is for the value of some variable measured for a group to be equal to zero. This could be the incidence of some disease, the number of 20- to 29-year-olds or, as in the above example, the prevalence of some serological marker in a group. If the frequency of a variable in our sample is 0%, what is the confidence interval for the 'true' value of this variable in the background population? It can hardly be a number below zero, but what is the upper limit?

The above formula is clearly not applicable when p is equal to zero (or when $p = 1$), since the entire value under the square root sign then becomes zero. Instead, we must use something called the binomial distribution in a rather backward fashion. The ordinary statistical question would be similar to the following: 'If we know that there are on average 5 elephants per square mile in this huge wildlife park, what is the chance that we shall not find any elephants at all if we search a randomly chosen square mile?' Here we want to know if we search a random sample of, say, 30 areas – each 1 mile square – of the wildlife park, and find no elephants at all, how high the average elephant density in the wildlife park could still be.

The amazing thing here is that when we observe zero cases in an unbiased, random sample from a larger population, the upper 95% confidence limit does not vary very much, regardless of the sample size. If we find zero cases of positive hepatitis A serology in a sample of 10 cases, the upper 95% confidence limit for the 'true' value of the seroprevalence in the background population is 3.1 per 10 cases, or 31%. If we obtain 0% seroprevalence in a sample of 1000 subjects, then the upper 95% confidence limit in the background population is 0.37% (3.69 cases divided by 1000). Remember the catch phrase 'The upper limit of 0 is around 3 to 4.' By this I mean that if you find no children with a BCG scar in a sample of n children (where n is at least 10) from a much larger population, then the upper 95% confidence interval for the prevalence of BCG scars in this population is 3 to 4 divided by n (closer to 3 for small samples, and up to 3.7 for large samples.)

This simple fact is not very well known in the medical world, and you will make quite an impression at departmental scientific meetings if you say something like 'Oh, you didn't find a single carrier of methicillin-resistant *Staphylococcus aureus* among the 200 health-care workers tested? This still means that the prevalence in the entire group could be some 1.5 to 2%' (you quickly do the calculation $3/200 \times 100$ or $4/200 \times 100$ in your head).

SIGNIFICANCE TESTING

It is becoming increasingly recognized by medical researchers and statisticians that the most informative way to indicate the statistical significance of a given value is to present the confidence interval as well. In the examples for

ORs and RRs in the previous chapters, two things are immediately obvious from a confidence interval.

1. If the 95% confidence interval does not include 1 (i.e. the entire interval is either above or below 1), then we know that there is a high probability that the risk factor studied is really associated with the disease, and that this is not just a chance finding.

2. The width of the confidence interval gives an indication of how precisely the OR or RR was measured in the study. If the 95% confidence interval for an RR was found to be from 1.3 to 15, then we would not really know whether this was a very important risk factor for the disease (high RR) or a relatively minor one.

However, much of medical literature still uses *significance tests* for these purposes, and in fact there are instances when confidence intervals are difficult to calculate and significance values can be obtained quite easily.

Probably the most common question behind all significance tests is the following. If one has just observed a difference between two groups of patients (one of the groups having, for example, higher haemoglobin values, a higher number of women, a lower attack rate, or longer incubation times), is this just something that has happened by chance, or does it point to a real difference between the groups?

The statistical theory underlying attempts to answer this question is quite complex in parts, and often in significance testing in real-life situations it is uncertain whether the necessary theoretical assumptions are met for such tests to be valid. Moreover, there is a good deal of philosophical argument as to what probabilities actually mean in this situation. The most important prerequisite is that the hypothesis you want to test should be stated *before* you perform the significance test. We shall refrain from going further into such discussions, but just point out here that for any variable measured in a group of people, there will be some type of random variation between the subjects. The above question then becomes phrased as follows. Is the difference observed between the groups just due to this variability, so that people who have a high value happened to end up in one group and people with a low value ended up in the other? Or would it be very unlikely that chance could divide a homogeneous group of people into two so apparently disparate groups?

Basically two different situations are possible.

1. We have measured the value of some continuous variable for all members in two groups. This could be their height, haemoglobin value, age, temperature, etc. All of these variables share in common the fact that they can assume, at least in principle, any value on a continuous line. This is not strictly true, because we would probably record height only in whole

centimetres, or temperature only in steps of 0.1°C, but theoretically they are continuous. For each of our two groups we could calculate an average value, and then compare them.

2. People are grouped into categories, such as exposed/unexposed, ill/healthy, men/women, older than/younger than, etc. We then look at our two groups of patients to see whether there are any differences between them in the proportions exposed/unexposed, ill/healthy, men/women, etc.

THE t-TEST

In the first situation described above with continuous data, one uses something called Student's *t*-test to determine whether there is a statistically significant difference between the two groups. Most basic statistics programs for a personal computer can do this very simply. One just enters the values for one of the patient groups in one column, and the values for the other group in the next column, and the programme delivers the probability (the *P-value*) that chance alone would cause a difference between the two groups as big as or bigger than the actually observed one. The lower the *P*- value, the less likely it is that this is a chance finding, and the more likely it is that there is a real difference between the groups.

The way to perform a *t*-test is as follows:

1. Call the groups 1 and 2. The numbers of subjects in the groups are called n_1 and n_2, respectively.

2. The average value for the first group (e.g. of the haemoglobin values) is called m_1, and for the second group is m_2.

3. Calculate the standard deviation of the values in the two groups separately. For the first group, subtract m_1, from each of the values, square these differences, and add all of the squares. Then divide this number by $(n_1 - 1)$, and take the square root of this number. The resulting figure is the standard deviation of the values in group 1, and is called s_1. Written in mathematics:

$$s_1 = \sqrt{\sum_1^n \frac{(x_1 - m_1)^2}{n_1 - 1}}$$

where x_i denotes all the individual measurements of the group. Then calculate s_2 in the same way.

The standard deviation is one way of describing how clustered the values in a group are around the average. A low standard deviation means that all of the values are grouped close to the mean, and a high standard deviation indicates that they are spread widely.

4. One also needs a combined standard deviation for both groups. This is called s_p, and is calculated as:

$$s_p^2 = \frac{(n_1 - 1)s_1^2 + (n_2 - 1)s_2^2}{n_1 + n_2 - 2}$$

5. The final figure we want is called t, and this is defined as:

$$t = \frac{m_1 - m_2}{s_p\sqrt{1/n_1 + 1/n_2}}$$

6. This t-value is then taken along to a ready-made table of ts, which is found at the back of most statistics textbooks. The actual significance levels vary according to the sizes of the two groups, but as a general rule of thumb, a t-value over about 2 means that there is a 5% chance or less that this difference between the two means would have arisen just by chance.

One can see that performing a t-test becomes quite laborious even for rather small samples. One should use a computer for this, and the above points are included primarily to demonstrate how it is actually being done.

However, two points are directly obvious. The higher the t-value, the lower the probability that the observed difference in averages between the groups is just a chance finding. From the last formula it can be seen that the greater the difference between the means, the higher the t-value will be. Furthermore, the smaller the combined measure of spread around the average values (s_p), the higher the t-value will be. A small difference between two groups may be quite significant if the standard deviations are low, whereas a large difference between two groups with high standard deviations might be just a chance finding.

There is one restriction on the usage of the t-test: if the standard deviations of the two groups are very different (e.g. if one is more than twice as great as the other), then the t-test should not be performed as described above. However, your favourite statistical computer program may have a valid test for the occasion, or else consult a statistician, since very different spreads in the two groups may mean that you should be interested in more than just comparing the two means.

THE CHI-SQUARED (χ^2) TEST

In the second of the two situations described above, we did not have continuous measurements of some variable for the two groups, but instead the numbers of people belonging to different categories. It then becomes rather bizarre to talk about the 'average sex' in a group of patients. The basic situation is just our old friend the 2×2 table, which could be for example as follows:

	III	Healthy	
Vaccinated	10	80	90
Non-vaccinated	40	20	60
	50	100	150

However, the 2×2 table could just as easily be extended to a table with more columns and/or rows if there were more categories of exposure or outcome, or both.

In this situation, the subjects could only belong to the two categories 'vaccinated' or 'non-vaccinated', and to either of the categories 'ill' or 'healthy'. There is no meaningful way of giving an average value for health in the vaccinated group, or an average vaccination status in the healthy group. This type of data is thus quite different to the t-test situation described above, and is usually termed categorical as opposed to continuous data.

In Chapter 5 we saw how to calculate an OR for such a table, and also a confidence interval for this value. If we now want to perform a significance test instead, we need to ask the following question. What is the probability that the 150 subjects of the study would divide this way into 'ill' and 'healthy' just by chance? A very low probability of such a chance arrangement would give increased weight to our hypothesis that the vaccine is effective.

The way to reason is as follows. There are 50 people who fall ill and 100 individuals who remain healthy. There are also 90 people who were vaccinated and 60 individuals who were not. All of these four numbers (the column and row sums, respectively) are given at the outset. If the vaccine was totally inefficient, we would assume that it did not matter whether or not one was vaccinated. Since one-third of the total group fell ill, this would be the expected proportion in each of the individual groups. In the vaccinated group of 90 people, we would expect 30 individuals to fall ill, and in the unvaccinated group of 60 subjects there should be 20 individuals who fall ill. The expected 2×2 table if the vaccine did not work at all would be as follows:

	III	Healthy	
Vaccinated	30	60	90
Non-vaccinated	20	40	60
	50	100	150

The general way of calculating the expected value for a cell in a 2×2 (or 3×3, or 5×3, etc.) table is to multiply the column sum at the bottom of the corresponding column by the row sum to the right, and to divide this number by the total in the lower right-hand corner. For the first cell in our example this would be $50 \times 90/150 = 30$, just as above. (In these calculations, one often obtains fractions of people in the cells of the expected table, but this does not affect the analysis at all.)

We can now compare the numbers in the expected table with the actual ones to see whether they are very different. One way is just to take the difference between the numbers in the corresponding cells (10 – 30 for the first cell, 80 – 60 for the second, and so on). If the vaccine had no effect, we would expect those differences to be small, and the larger they are, the more the result of our study deviates from what would be expected by chance distribution of the cases. The χ^2 test now involves squaring all of these differences, dividing each square by its expected value (from the table above), and then adding them. The higher this number, the less likely it is that the distribution of ill and healthy subjects according to vaccination status could have occurred just by chance. For a 2×2 table like this, a χ^2 value above 3.84 indicates that there is less than a 5% probability that the result occurred by chance.

In the above example, the calculation would be as follows:

$$\chi^2 = \frac{(10 - 30)^2}{30} + \frac{(40 - 20)^2}{20} + \frac{(80 - 60)^2}{60} + \frac{(20 - 40)^2}{40} = 50$$

We can see that there is a very small probability indeed that this high χ^2 value would arise by chance, and we can state that there is statistical support for the hypothesis that the vaccine does have a protective effect. In fact, the probability that this would be a chance finding can be calculated to be $P < 0.0001$.

When you look up a χ^2 table, you will find that it mentions something called 'degrees of freedom'. For tables such as the one above, this is concerned with the numbers of rows and columns (categories for exposure and outcome). The number of degrees of freedom is equal to (number of rows – 1) multiplied by (number of columns – 1), and thus for a 2×2 table it is $(2 - 1) \times (2 - 1) = 1$. For a 3×4 table (three different outcomes and four different exposures), there would be $(3 - 1) \times (4 - 1) = 6$ degrees of freedom, and you would have to refer to this table for the χ^2 test. (Degrees of freedom are often abbreviated to df.)

A quick way to calculate the χ^2 value from the general 2×2 table from Chapter 5

	Cases	Controls	
Exposed	a	b	a + b
Not exposed	c	d	c + d
	a + c	b + d	N

is with the following formula:

$$\chi^2 = \frac{(ad - bc)^2 \times n}{(a + c)(b + d)(a + b)(c + d)}$$

where the parentheses in the denominator are just the column and row sums.

Since the χ^2 test is so easy to perform, it can often be used for an initial check even for continuous data, where one would otherwise use the t-test. For example, if one wants to compare temperatures in two groups of patients, one could just choose a value that seems to be somewhere in the middle of all of the temperature readings from both groups, and count the number of subjects in each group who have a temperature above or below this value. The four figures thus obtained are entered into a 2×2 table, and the χ^2 value is calculated. If this χ^2 figure yields a low P-value, then you can be quite confident that the t-test will also yield a low P-value.

An approximate estimate for a 2×2 table is that the χ^2 value should be above 4 for the difference to be statistically significant at the 5% level.

There are some important restrictions on when the χ^2 test can be used. It is an approximate method that becomes increasingly valid the larger the size of the study. As a general rule of thumb these restrictions are as follows.

1. Either the total sample size (n above) should be greater than 40, or

2. n could be between 20 and 40, but none of the *expected* values in the 2×2 table should be less than 5.

If neither of these conditions is fulfilled, one must use Fisher's exact test, which is the subject of the next section.

FISHER'S EXACT TEST

This test is a favourite with medical researchers, perhaps partly because of the word 'exact' in the name of the test. It builds on the same general idea as the two tests described above. In other words, what is the chance/probability that the pattern of outcomes we have observed would arise just by chance? Fisher's test is mainly used for 2×2 tables in which the individual values are too small for a χ^2 test to be allowed.

If we have a 2×2 table with small numbers that appears as follows:

	Cases	Controls	
Exposed	8	3	11
Unexposed	2	5	7
	10	8	18

we cannot use the χ^2 test, nor can we use the formula for the confidence interval of an OR from Chapter 5. The concept underlying Fisher's test is the following. In this study we had 10 cases and 8 controls. In total, 11 subjects were exposed and 7 subjects were not exposed. These four figures make up the column and row sums, respectively. Keeping these sums constant, in how many different ways could the 18 subjects of the study be distributed on the four different cells? Two other possibilities would be as follows:

	Cases	Controls	
Exposed	7	4	11
Unexposed	3	4	7
	10	8	18

and

	Cases	Controls	
Exposed	9	2	11
Unexposed	1	6	7
	10	8	18

and there are obviously several other possible distributions. The probability of getting any given 2×2 table when the row and column sums are fixed can be shown to be as follows:

$$\frac{(a + c)!(b + d)!(a + b)!(c + d)!}{a!\; b!\; c!\; d!\; n!}$$

where a, b, c and d are the four cells as usual. The exclamation mark stands for 'factorial', and $a!$ is defined as multiplying a with all of the integers less than a down to 1. The symbol $6!$ thus means $6 \times 5 \times 4 \times 3 \times 2 \times 1 = 720$. (By definition $0! = 1$.)

Using this formula, we can calculate the probability of getting the first 2×2 table of this section as follows:

$$\frac{10! \times 8! \times 11! \times 7!}{8! \times 3! \times 2! \times 5! \times 18!} = 0.08.$$

However, we are not interested only in the probability of this distribution, but also in the chance of getting an even more extreme result from a random spread of the 18 subjects. 'Extreme' here means an even greater difference in the proportion exposed among the cases and the controls. The third 2×2 table above would thus be more extreme than the original one, and the most extreme distribution which would still conform to our fixed row and column totals would be as follows:

	Cases	Controls	
Exposed	10	1	11
Unexposed	0	7	7
	10	8	18

where there were no unexposed individuals at all among the cases, and only one exposed subject among the eight controls.

In calculating the P-value for a distribution of cases according to Fisher's test, we add the probability for the observed distribution to the probabilities for all of the more extreme distributions possible. In this example the probabilities for the two more extreme distributions can be calculated to be 0.009 and 0.0003, respectively, with the above formula. The P-value would be $0.08 + 0.009 + 0.0003 = 0.09$, and it would thus be quite likely that we would obtain the observed distribution at the top of this section just by chance.

Even for very low numbers in the 2×2 table, Fisher's test becomes very time-consuming to perform, and the use of a standard statistics computer program is strongly recommended.

ONE-SIDED AND TWO-SIDED TESTING

An additional issue in significance testing is whether one should perform so-called one-sided or two-sided tests. Again this is a somewhat philosophical discussion, and it really depends on the assumptions that one makes before performing the test. The basic hypothesis (often called the *null hypothesis*) in the three statistical methods described above is always that there is no real difference between the groups, and that the observed difference is a random effect. We then proceed to calculate the probability that this difference would arise at random, and if this probability is very small, we deduce that it is unlikely that we have made a chance finding.

If we have no a priori idea about the direction of the difference between the groups (e.g. it is just as plausible that the average temperature in group A will be higher than that in group B as the other way round), then we should perform a two-sided test. This will tell us the added probabilities of observing as large a difference, or a larger one, in the mean temperature of A − B and of observing the same difference for B − A.

However, if we have some previous knowledge that treatment C is at least as good as treatment D, and possibly better, then we are only interested in finding out whether the patients who receive treatment C fare significantly better than those on treatment D. In this instance we could perform a one-sided test of significance, which would tell us the probability that the patients on treatment C fared as well as or better than the patients on treatment D just by chance.

The χ^2 test is always two-sided and thus does not differ with regard to the ways in which the observed difference may go. Tables for the *t*-test include columns for both one-sided and two-sided tests, whereas Fisher's test as described above is one-sided. One simple approximation to make the *P*-value given by Fisher's test apply to a two-sided situation is just to double it.

It may be tempting to choose the *p*-value for the one-sided test from a *t*-table, since it is always lower than the two-sided one, but this can only be done if one has firm prior knowledge that the observed difference can only go in one direction. In a test of a new drug, it would be just as important to find out that it was actually detrimental to the patients as to ascertain that it was beneficial, and our test must include both of these possibilities.

GENERAL NOTES ON SIGNIFICANCE TESTS

Like all of the concepts borrowed by epidemiology from statistical theory, significance tests assume unbiased sampling. A *p*-value only tells us the probability that the difference we have observed is due to chance and random effects. If there was a bias in the selection of subjects, or in the type of exposure between the groups, or in the measurement of outcomes, the *p*-value will tell us nothing about the precision or validity of our findings.

There are two common misconceptions in the interpretation of *P*-values. The first assumes that a low or very low *P*-value 'proves' that the difference we have found is due to the treatment, or to the exposure, etc. Statistical hypothesis testing by significance analysis never proves anything – it merely tells us that the probability that our observed effect should be due to chance is low. If one wants to be very cautious, one should thus state the findings as follows: 'statistical significance testing gives an indication that the observed finding is not merely due to chance.'

Continuing this line of reasoning, one should remember that many articles in the medical literature regard a *P*-value of less than 5% as significant. This is equivalent to stating that there is only one chance in 20 that the result was due to chance. Strictly interpreted, this means that out of 20 such studies reporting significant associations, one will just be a chance finding. With the large volume of scientific medical articles being published each month, the number that report spurious findings as facts is thus hardly negligible.

The second misconception works in the opposite way. If the outcome of a study is found not to be statistically significant, this is sometimes reported as follows: 'there is no association between exposure A and outcome B'. This may be completely wrong, and there may be quite a strong association, although the study failed to confirm it. Mostly, this is due to too small a sample size, and a similar study on a larger number of subjects may well reveal significant differences. A lack of significance in a test does not prove that the opposite is true.

Finally, just a paragraph about the word 'significance'. This is a word with many positive connotations, but one should always remember that it only addresses statistical significance. A very significant statistical finding may have a very low clinical significance. Studies may show a significantly increased risk of developing Hodgkin's disease after tonsillectomy in puberty, but the risk to the individual is so small anyway that even a doubling may be personally insignificant, since the vast majority of people who have had a tonsillectomy will not develop this lymphoma. Not even for differential diagnosis in patients with prolonged fever will the fact that the patient has had a tonsillectomy be of much assistance. The clinical significance of such a finding would be low.

ESTIMATING SAMPLE SIZE

Probably the most common question I am asked by colleagues who want to perform some kind of study is 'How many patients do I need?'. This is not a very easy question to answer, partly because my immediate response is always 'For what?', and partly because the requirements for an answer are quite strict.

The first thing one needs to consider is how small any difference between the two groups could be and still be clinically interesting. In a clinical trial, how much better must the patients on the new drug fare (as measured by the number of days in hospital, incidence of adverse reactions, number of hepatitis C RNA copies/mL of blood, or as percentage protected by a vaccine) for you to think that the results of a study would be useful? If it could be shown that a new antibiotic for sore throat shortened the time with fever > 37.0°C from 2.3 to 2.2 days, would you be very enthusiastic? Or if in an epidemiological study it could be shown that some risk factor increased the attack rate of a certain infection from 45% to 47%, could you suppress a yawn?

Thus one has to state firmly something like 'If this exposure gives an OR of 1.5 or higher for disease, I want to be able to find that in my study, but an OR below 1.5 is of little clinical relevance, and in that case I don't care.' However, you will find that in real life there are surprisingly few researchers who are able to formulate their research questions so precisely.

In the absence of such clear ideas of what one wants to achieve, one should at least be able to guess how high the OR from the study will be.

The second thing one needs to know is the incidence (or prevalence) of the exposure that one wants to study in the background population (e.g. among the controls in a case-control study). This means that in order to calculate the necessary sample size for a case-control study, one must have some prior knowledge of how common an exposure is among non-cases. One will therefore often have to make a pre-study before one embarks on the originally intended study. In a clinical trial situation, one would have to know the outcome in patients on placebo (or on the best available previous treatment) before one could calculate a sample size.

Thirdly, one must judge how much risk one is willing to accept that the study will fail to identify a difference between the groups even though there is one. This figure subtracted from 100% is called the *power* of the study. A power close to 100% means that there is very little risk that we shall miss a truly existing difference. A power of 65% means that there is a 35% risk that our study will fail to find a truly existing association between exposure and outcome.

Fourthly, one must decide what significance level one wishes to attach to the association (OR, RR or percentage difference) one finds in the study. Should one call a *P*-value below 5% or below 1% significant?

In most instances, people settle for a power of 80% (which means that there is only a 20% risk that a real association will be missed), and for a significance level of 5% (as always).

Fifthly, one must choose which statistical test one will use to analyse the data after the study has been conducted.

For a case–control study in which one decides to use a χ^2 test to analyse the data after the study, one would calculate the sample size as follows (assuming an equal number of cases and controls).

1. Make an educated guess about the OR that the study will yield for a certain exposure (or define the smallest OR that is of any clinical interest).

2. Estimate what proportion of the controls have the exposure in question. Call this π_1.

3. Calculate an auxiliary variable called π_2 from the following formula:

$$\pi_2 = OR \times \pi_1/(1 - \pi_1 + OR \times \pi_1)$$

4. Call the average of π_1 and π_2, $(\pi_1 + \pi_2)/2 = \pi_m$

5. The number of subjects needed in each group (if the significance level is 5% and power is 80%) is then:

$$m = 1.96 \sqrt{2\,\pi_m\,(1 - \pi_m)} + 0.84 \sqrt{\frac{(\pi_1\,(1 - \pi_1) + \pi_2\,(1 - \pi_2))^2}{(\pi_2 - \pi_2)^2}}$$

Quite a mouthful, wouldn't you agree? However, there are computer programs to do this (EpiInfo has an easy-to-use module). These programs also allow you to try different values for significance and power, as well as different numbers of controls per case.

If you want the power to detect a true difference to be 90%, exchange 0.84 in the formula for 1.28. If you want to be certain at the 1% level, exchange 1.96 for 2.58.

For example, suppose we wanted to show that mosquito bites are a risk factor for tularaemia by performing a case–control study. We guess that the OR for having been exposed to a mosquito bite if one has tularaemia is 2. Since the normal incubation period is 3–5 days, we shall ask the controls about bites in the last week, and we shall assume that 30% will answer yes. π_1 is thus 0.3.

How many subjects do we need?

First, we calculate $\pi_2 = 2 \times 0.3/(1 - 0.3 + 2 \times 0.3) = 0.46$.

Then $\pi_m = (0.46 + 0.3)\,2 = 0.38$.

With 5% significance and 90% power we obtain the following:

$$m = 1.96 \sqrt{2 \times 0.38 \times 0.62} + 1.28 \sqrt{\frac{(0.3 \times 0.7 + 0.46 \times 0.54)^2}{(0.46 - 0.30)^2}} = 191$$

When calculating sample size, it is always safer to round upwards, and we would thus estimate that we will need 200 cases and 200 controls for this study.

Personally, I am very sceptical about sample size calculations. As is evident from the above, they almost require that one has done the study first, since OR and proportion exposed among controls must be known. Moreover, the exact numbers that come out of the calculations give an unjustified impression of reliability. They can be useful if one wants a rough approximation of the numbers needed (e.g. 'Do I need 5000 subjects, or would 1000 suffice?'), and they should always be generously rounded upwards.

If instead of an OR in a case–control study you want to calculate the sample size necessary to compare two proportions more correctly than in the rule of thumb at the beginning of this chapter, you just start from point 4 above with π_1 and π_2 as the two proportions.

The smallest sample size possible

If you are completely convinced that you have found an exposure that is completely associated with outcome, you could demonstrate this on a 5% significance level with a sample of just 4 cases and 4 controls. The 2×2 table would be as follows:

	Cases	Controls	
Exposed	4	0	4
Unexposed	0	4	4
	4	4	8

Fisher's test gives a *P*-value for this table (just this one, there is none more extreme with 8 subjects) to be 4! 4!/8! = 1/70 one-sided, or 1/35 = 2.9% two-sided. Just remember that the choice of cases and controls should be completely unbiased . . .

SUMMARY

If we study a sample of subjects from a larger population, there will always be a chance component with regard to which subjects we happen to choose. The proportion in our sample with disease A may have become higher than the proportion in the background population, or the proportion in our sample with antibody to disease B may be lower than that in the general population. Statistical theory tells us how different our sample is likely to be from the total population, and it expresses this by assigning confidence intervals to figures estimated from the sample that tell us which values are likely for these figures in the total population.

If we find a large difference between two study groups, either in some continuous variable such as haemoglobin value or age, or in the proportion of subjects with different characteristics, we could calculate the probability that the difference would have arisen by chance. For continuous variables this is done with the *t*-test, and for categorical variables with the χ^2 test. If the numbers of a 2×2 table are small, Fisher's test gives a better alternative to χ^2 tests.

As a general rule of thumb, a *t*-value greater than 2, and a χ^2 value for a 2×2 table greater than 4 indicate that the finding is statistically significant at the 5% level.

A finding that is statistically very significant could well be of little clinical significance.

Sample size calculations require much prior knowledge about the problem to be of much use.

Chapter 8
Clinical epidemiology: sensitivity, specificity and misclassification

Here we discuss how well we measure the things we want to study. A test is characterized by its sensitivity and specificity, but one also has to consider the context in which the test will be used. When measurement is imprecise, we shall place subjects in the wrong groups, which is called misclassification, and might have serious consequences.

SENSITIVITY AND SPECIFICITY

In order to make a diagnosis, we interview the patient, conduct a physical examination, and we may perform tests or investigations. For each of these steps certain findings will indicate that the patient has a certain disease – with greater or lesser probability. Likewise, we know that the absence of certain findings may indicate that the patient does not have the disease. The two main terms used to describe how well a test performs are *sensitivity* and *specificity*. These two terms are rather unfortunate, partly because they are too similar and partly because they do not give any intuitive feeling for what they mean.

Sensitivity measures how often a test turns out positive when it is being used on people who we (in some other way) know to have the disease. For example, if one takes a cervical chlamydial sample for culture from 100 women with chlamydia infection, the culture will be positive in 80 of them at most, the test method is simply not perfect. In this case we say that the sensitivity of chlamydia culture is 80%.

Another example is the culture of stools for salmonella. In asymptomatic carriers, the sensitivity of one faecal culture is only around 70%. By taking a second sample, we shall obtain a positive culture from some of those who were negative the first time, and by taking a third sample we may find salmonella in some of the remainder. By counting all of the people who have at least one positive culture, the sensitivity could be increased to over 90%. This is the reason for using repeated cultures when looking for salmonella carriers.

An example of a test with low sensitivity is blood culture from patients with agranulocytosis and suspected bacteraemia. Pathogens are seldom found, but in most cases one nevertheless chooses to treat with antibiotics just on the basis of suspicion of bacteraemia.

Note that the definition of sensitivity implies that there is a *gold standard* (or 'truth') somewhere – there must be another way to decide unambiguously whether or not the patient has the disease. As you are surely aware, there are not many diseases for which this is true, and sensitivity is thus a somewhat abstract measure. Most often sensitivity is actually being measured against the best available previous test.

Specificity is rather the reverse, it tells how often the test turns out negative when it is being used on people who we know do *not* have the disease. Ideally, a test for a disease should always be negative when used on healthy individuals, and such a test would be said to have a specificity of 100%. For example, before it became possible to test for infection with hepatitis C in prospective blood donors, some blood banks used a raised alanine-amino-transferase (ALT) value as a marker of possible hepatitis. However, if this test was applied to a large group of donors, this group would include several who had elevated ALT values for other reasons, but who would be excluded from donating blood because they would be suspected of having hepatitis. This particular test would have a specificity well below 100% in the diagnosis of hepatitis. This lack of specificity may not be a great problem for the blood bank, because other donors could be found, but it may create problems for the excluded donors who are told that they may have infectious hepatitis.

Low sensitivity means that the test will miss a lot of individuals who have the disease, whereas low specificity implies that the test will put many people in the 'disease group' who do not have the disease. In epidemiological jargon, one often says that a test with poor sensitivity will give rise to a lot of 'false negatives', whereas one with poor specificity will yield many 'false positives'.

Few tests used in medicine have a specificity of more than 99%, but an example of the importance of high specificity comes from the use of HIV tests. If we tested 500 000 blood donors for HIV infection each year with an antibody test having 'only' 99% specificity, we would label 5000 positive, even if there was not a single case of 'true' HIV infection in the group. In reality, things are not that bad, as the specificity of the present HIV antibody tests is only some tenths of a per cent below 100%, and all positive results are verified with Western blots, which means that the problem with false positives is negligible.

An example of a test with low specificity is the use of nasopharyngeal culture to decide whether or not a child with a runny nose should be given antibiotics. Many children carry *Haemophilus influenzae* or *Branhamella catarrhalis* behind their noses without needing any treatment with antibiotics, and the result of the test would not guide our decision very much.

For most tests there is a conflict between demands for high sensitivity and high specificity. A good example comes from the use of serology to decide whether or not a patient has had an infection. For such a test one needs a cut-off point at a certain antibody titre, so that those who have higher values will be said to have had the disease in question, whereas those with lower titres are said not to have had it. If this cut-off value is set very low, one will not miss any of those with a previous infection (high sensitivity), but one will also include a number of individuals who only have unspecific reactions to the test, without any real markers (low specificity). If one instead raises the cut-off point, one will not label anyone with unspecific reaction as positive (high specificity), but instead a number of patients who have true low levels of markers of past infection will be missed (low sensitivity). We shall return to the question of cut-off points in Chapter 16 on seroepidemiology.

Although the words *sensitivity* and *specificity* are most often employed in connection with laboratory tests, it is quite useful to think in those terms as well when interviewing a patient or performing a physical examination. The presence of Koplik's spots on the inside of the cheek of a child diagnoses measles with a very high specificity (it cannot be anything else), whereas cough in the same child diagnoses measles with a very high sensitivity ('Without cough, no measles', as my old professor used to say – even if this criterion will also include many children who do not have measles, which means low specificity).

It is also worthwhile pondering the high diagnostic specificity of the first moments of your contact with a patient. An unknown patient waiting outside your office door could have any one of thousands of diseases. As soon as he or she comes in through the door, at least 50% of these become implausible, as you see the patient's gender, approximate age, gait and general appearance. After the first minute of discussion with the patient, you are probably down to at most 10 possible diagnoses.

We seldom pause to think about the enormous speed at which this diagnostic process occurs, excluding 99% of all diagnoses in next to no time, and leaving a very small number for more elaborate tests and procedures. It could be described as a chain of unconscious 'tests' whereby we confidently exclude diagnoses with a very high specificity.

TWO EXAMPLES

Fever and malaria

A study from Malawi attempted to assess the sensitivity and specificity of directly observable clinical signs for the diagnosis of malaria and pneumonia in children.[1]

The study subjects were 1469 children under 5 years of age who came to a children's outpatient department with fever and/or cough. The purely clinical definition of malaria was as follows:

- fever or history of fever;

and the definition of pneumonia was as follows:

- history of cough; or

- difficulty in breathing and lower chest-wall indrawing; or

- increased respiratory rate.

Blood films for microscopic examination for malaria parasites were taken from all of the children, but only those with evidence of pneumonia (or who had parasitaemia) had a chest X-ray.

A total of 1290 children fulfilled the clinical definition of malaria (i.e. fever or history of fever). Of these, 486 children had a positive blood film, while in 804 children no parasitaemia could be diagnosed. In total, 179 children did not meet the clinical case definition, but of these 22 individuals had a positive blood film.

If we assume that 'positive blood film' is the gold standard for diagnosing malaria, we would say that our clinical case definition has correctly diagnosed 486 of the 486 + 22 = 508, truly infected children. The sensitivity of the clinical definition will thus be as follows:

$$\text{sensitivity} = \frac{486}{508} = 96\%$$

which means that out of all the truly infected children this crude 'test' will identify almost everyone.

On the other hand, only 179 − 22 = 157 of the children who had a negative blood film for malaria were correctly labelled negative by the clinical definition. There were also 804 children who were positive according to the clinical malaria definition, but who were negative according to their blood films. The total number of true negatives was thus 804 + 157 = 961, and the specificity of the clinical definition is as follows:

$$\text{specificity} = \frac{157}{961} = 16\%$$

This means that five out of six children who did not have malaria would still be diagnosed as having the disease according to the clinical definition.

Stated in words, what we have found is that almost all cases of malaria will have or have had fever, but that many cases of fever will not be due to malaria.

Since children without clinical symptoms of pneumonia did not have X-rays taken, we have no 'gold standard' for this disease and cannot calculate the sensitivity or specificity of the above three clinical signs for the diagnosis of pneumonia.

Smell and streptococcal infection

In the absence of microbiological results, the diagnosis of streptococcal infection in patients who present with a sore throat is often difficult. Erythema of the tonsils, exudate, and painful cervical lymph nodes are used to make a clinical diagnosis. A study in four general practices in Israel tried to assess whether the doctor's nose could also be used as a diagnostic device[2].

The doctors were asked to smell the breath of 105 consecutive patients presenting with fever and sore throat. If the breath was putrid, this was regarded as an indication of streptococcal infection. All of the patients then had throat swabs taken for streptococcal culture.

In total, 40 patients were culture positive, and the smell test diagnosed 24 of these individuals. A total of 65 patients were culture negative, but nine of these were judged to have putrid breath.

The sensitivity of this smell test is thus 24/40 = 60%, and the specificity is 56/65 = 86%. The absence of a putrid smell is thus a rather good indication that the patient does not have a streptococcal infection (and should thus probably not receive any antibiotics).

POSITIVE PREDICTIVE VALUE

This is a very important concept, but it is frequently overlooked when the merits of different tests are being discussed. It is concerned with the environment in which the test is being used – the same test might be useful in one setting and have a limited value in another. Whereas a test for haematuria might diagnose schistosomiasis infection with high probability in a region in Africa, it would not serve this purpose in Europe, where the prevalence of this infection is low, and most cases of haematuria are due to other causes.

If a test has 100% sensitivity and 100% specificity, it does not matter where one uses it – it will correctly label everyone tested. However, when these values (as they always do) lie below 100%, the actual prevalence of the disease one is testing for becomes important. The problem arises from the way in which one should interpret a result of the test.

Let us assume that we have an HIV antibody test with 99.9% sensitivity and 99.5% specificity and that we do not have access to Western blots. We want to use the test to determine the HIV prevalence in a population of 10 000, where the true prevalence (unknown to us) is 10%. (Again, note the abstract nature of discussions on sensitivity and specificity: how can we know that the prevalence is 10% before we have measured it? As in the comments about 'true' ORs in Chapter 4, we must assume that in the world of Plato there does exist a value for the prevalence in the group and that this value is known at least to God.)

Thus there must be 1000 seropositive individuals in this population, and since our test has 99.9% sensitivity, it will correctly label 999 of these subjects as infected. One infected individual will not be diagnosed. There are also 9000 seronegative subjects, and with the given specificity (99.5%),

$0.995 \times 9000 = 8955$ of these will be labelled as negative. However, our test will also yield 45 false positives.

The *positive predictive value* (PPV) is the proportion of all those who test positive who really are infected. In this case $999 + 45 = 1044$ individuals will have a positive test, but we know that only 999 of those subjects are really infected:

$$PPV = \frac{999}{999+45} = \frac{999}{1044} = 0.957, \text{ or } 96\%$$

This means that for someone with a positive test result, there is a 96% probability that they really are infected, which explains the term positive predictive value.

Now let us use the same test in another population of 10 000 subjects, where the true (equally mysteriously known) prevalence is 1/1000.

Thus there are 10 seropositive individuals, and our test will correctly identify all of them. There are also 9990 seronegative individuals, and of these $0.995 \times 9990 = 9940$ subjects will have a negative test result. However, 50 individuals will be false positives. In this case the positive predictive value will be as follows:

$$PPV = \frac{10}{10+50} = \frac{10}{60} = 0.166, \text{ or } 17\%$$

In this second population, a person who tests positive will thus have only a 17% chance of being truly infected, whereas 83% of those whom the test labels as positive are in reality seronegative. It is clear that even this exceedingly good test becomes quite useless in this population.

(One might argue that it is not much more fun to be mislabelled positive in a high-prevalence population than in a low-prevalence one, and that the number of false positives is about equal in the two cases. This is a valid point, but for diagnostic purposes, and even more so for epidemiological ones, there is a large difference in the applicability of the test in the two situations. If you were to give someone treatment on the basis of the results of only one test like this, you would feel a great deal better if you knew that there was a strong chance that they really had the disease.)

The simplest way to think about the PPV is to look at the specificity of the test, and to see what percentage of the population will be false positive. This number will be the same in all populations, regardless of the true prevalence. One then considers the expected prevalence, to see whether it is considerably higher than the false-positive portion. If it is, one can disregard the false positives, and the test will be useful. This simplified way of looking at the PPV arises from the fact that most laboratory tests have a sensitivity of at least 90%, and then the specificity becomes much more crucial for the PPV.

In the malaria example given above, the PPV for the clinical definition would have been 486/1290 = 38%. Obviously, this value would have been even lower in a setting where malaria was less common.

When a new test has been developed, its sensitivity and specificity have often been measured under ideal circumstances, with much attention paid to technical detail, and a high-prevalence group of samples for evaluation. As the test enters clinical medicine, it often performs less well. This is due to a number of factors ranging from less experienced staff to a lower overall prevalence in the population being tested.

A NEW 2 × 2 TABLE

All of the above terms can be nicely defined using our old friend, the 2 × 2 table. It looks much the same as before, but the rows and columns are named differently:

	Have disease	**Healthy**	
Test positive	a	b	$a + b$
Test negative	c	d	$c + d$
	$a + c$	$b + d$	

In a perfect test, c and b are both equal to 0, since only those who are ill test positive and only those who are healthy test negative.

The definitions of our terms are as follows:

$$\text{sensitivity} = \frac{a}{a + c}$$

$$\text{specificity} = \frac{d}{d + b}$$

$$\text{PPV} = \frac{a}{a + b}$$

and there is also something called *negative predictive value* (NPV), defined as

$$\text{NPV} = \frac{d}{d + c}$$

which is the reverse of the PPV (i.e. the proportion of truly healthy individuals out of all those with a negative test).

Personally, I always find all of these definitions impossible to remember, and I have to look them up every time I need them. It might be a good idea for you to fold the top corner of this page ('a dog's ear'), so that you will know where to look for this schematic 2 × 2 table in the future.

As was pointed out above, we should probably be thinking more in terms of sensitivity and specificity with regard to the questions we use when we are interviewing a patient, or the physical examinations that we perform. There is a lot of historical deadwood here, and much of it arguably adds very little to the diagnostic process.

RELIABILITY

This term describes how 'constant' a test is (i.e. whether it will give the same value if used repeatedly on the same sample). We would not want it to give different answers at different times. Also, will the test yield the same result in different laboratories? Another term is that the test should be *reproducible*. High reliability is mostly a problem for laboratory staff, but even when clinical measurements are involved, reliability can be improved by letting several independent doctors judge a specific finding.

VALIDITY

This is a more subtle concept than reliability, and it is concerned with the question of whether we really measure what we want to know. Using the presence or absence of a high sedimentation rate to decide which patients have a bacterial infection (and should therefore be given antibiotics) is not a very valid test. A test for 14-3-3 protein in cerebrospinal fluid does not really identify any particular prion – it is just a marker of neural damage.

A test may be perfectly reliable, giving quite dependable values each time, but may still not tell us what we want to know about the patient's disease. If the association between the test result and 'true' disease in the patient is weak, then this test would not be very valid for the situation in which we apply it.

MISCLASSIFICATION

In the discussions of risks, RRs, ORs and rate ratios in the previous chapters, we assumed that all study subjects were assigned to the correct groups (e.g. with regard to what they were exposed to or what happened to them).

One exception to this occurs in the very first example in Chapter 4, where one of the guests at the dinner could have forgotten what he ate (uncertain exposure). Another occurred in the discussion of biases in connection with the person-year graph in Chapter 6, where it was pointed out that if the subjects that we designed as 'losses to follow-up' really had died (uncertain outcome), this would underestimate the rate.

It has been stated that good epidemiology is really a question of accurate measurements. If the subjects are somehow classified in the wrong group, this is called misclassification. There are two types, namely random and non-random misclassification.

Random misclassification

This is the lesser of the two problems. It occurs when our methods of measuring risk factors or disease are less than perfect, as they almost always are. Let us consider an example.

In a case–control study in Gothenburg,[3] 5741 young women were tested for chlamydia infection, and at the same time were asked about certain risk factors for being infected. One such 'risk factor' that was studied was the duration of their present sexual relationship. The women who had no partner or whose present relationship had lasted less than 1 year were compared with those who had had a steady sexual partner for more than 1 year. The actual 2×2 table for this factor was as follows:

	Chlamydia positive	Chlamydia negative	
Present relationship ≤ 1 year	280	2408	2688
Present relationship > 1 year	144	2909	3053
	424	5317	5741

From this table we can see that the OR for the exposure 'no or short relationship' if one was infected with chlamydia was (280/144)/(2408/2909) = 2.35. Since the disease was relatively rare in this population (overall prevalence less than 10%), one could interpret this as an apparently lower risk of being infected with chlamydia if one has a longer, steady relationship, which seems plausible.

However, we learned from the above discussion about sensitivity that a chlamydia culture only correctly identifies 80% of the infected cases. This means that we have missed 20% of the cases. The true total number of infected cases should not have been 424 as in the 2×2 table, but 25% more, i.e. 530. How should these extra 106 cases be divided between the two groups of women?

Obviously there must be an equal chance of being a false negative whether one has had a short relationship or a long one, as the length of the relationship can hardly affect the sensitivity of the test. This is just what we mean by random misclassification – it affects both groups in the same way. Thus the number of infected cases in both groups should really increase by 25%. In the short-relationship group, 25% × 280 = 70 more of those labelled negative should have been positive, and in the long-relationship group, 25% × 180 = 36 truly positive cases were not diagnosed.

The specificity of a chlamydia culture is 100% for all practical purposes, so there are no false positives. The 'true' 2×2 table would thus have been as follows:

	Chlamydia positive	Chlamydia negative	
Present relationship ≤ 1 year	350	2338	2688
Present relationship > 1 year	180	2873	3053
	530	5211	5741

where we have added 70 positive cases to the short-relationship group (and taken away 70 negatives), and moved 36 women from the negative square to the positive one in the long-relationship group.

The OR for this table would be (350/180)/(2338/2873) = 2.39, or slightly higher than the value of 2.35 given above. This difference may not be very impressive, but the exercise points to the main feature of random misclassification, namely that *it reduces the strength of the associations found in an epidemiological study.* The association betwen length of relationship and chlamydia infection actually becomes somewhat stronger when misclassification is accounted for. Random misclassification will never create a bias that makes a factor seem significant for development of disease, but it may well decrease the true value of an OR or an RR, so that they no longer seem to be significant. In our example, the less than total sensitivity of the test for chlamydia makes the OR seem slightly lower than it should have been.

This misclassification was about disease vs. no disease, but the same reasoning would apply if exposure had been randomly misclassified. In this example, exposure could have been misclassified if, for example, a certain proportion of the women who reported long relationships had really had short ones, and vice versa. Such random misclassification would also have rendered the OR too low.

Non-random (or preferential) misclassification

This is a much more serious problem, and a bias introduced by non-random misclassification could really go any way. It occurs when exposure status influences the assignment to cases and controls, or the other way round – when disease status influences the assignment to exposure groups.

An example of the first type of non-random misclassification would be the following. Suppose that one wishes to study how risk factors for HIV infection in children vary with age. If a simple serological test is used, the performance of the test will vary with exposure (age in this case), since very young children might just have passively transmitted antibodies from their mothers.

An example of the latter type of non-random misclassification comes from a study of risk factors for hepatitis C infection. Blood donors who were found to be positive for hepatitis C were interviewed extensively in the clinic about possible exposures. The controls were blood donors without signs of hepatitis C infection who were interviewed by telephone. It is easy to envisage that it would be much more difficult to press the latter about socially sensitive transmission routes such as illicit drug use or sexual behaviour. Such a study might easily lead to non-random misclassification of exposures.

Non-random misclassification is really just another name for the different types of biases that were discussed at the end of Chapter 6 and, just like these, it can often be eliminated by careful clinical consideration.

SUMMARY

Epidemiology is very much concerned with good measurements. If the outcome of a study is whether or not the patient dies, or if the risk factor studied is gender, this is usually a small problem, but as soon as we use some type of test to measure exposure or outcome, bias may be introduced.

The ability of a test to detect the truly diseased individuals in a population is called sensitivity, whereas its ability to select the healthy ones is called specificity. The usefulness of a test depends not only on these two parameters, but also on the prevalence of the disease in the population, and the three together define the positive predictive value.

Random misclassification can weaken an association, even to the point where a significant difference becomes insignificant, but it can never create significant findings. Preferential misclassification is just another name for bias, and might work in any way in a study, non-significant associations becoming significant, and vice versa.

REFERENCES

1. Redd SC, Bloland PB, Kazembe PN, Patrick E, Tembenu R, Campbell CC. Usefulness of clinical case-definition in guiding therapy for African children with malaria or pneumonia. *Lancet* 1992; **340**: 1140–43.

2. Nakar S, Kahan E, Weingarten M. Can you smell the strep? *Lancet* 1994; **343**: 729–30.

3. Ramstedt K, Forssman L, Giesecke J, Granath F. Risk factors for *Chlamydia trachomatis* infection in 6810 young women attending family planning clinics. *Int J STD AIDS* 1992; **3**: 117–22.

Chapter 9
Multivariate analysis
and interaction

This chapter discusses the simultaneous analysis of several risk factors. The procedure of stratification is explained, and the Mantel–Haenszel algorithm for calculating an adjusted RR or OR is described. The ideas behind matching receive a mention, and the 2 × 2 table for matched studies is demonstrated. There is also a short introduction to the concept of regression models, and finally interaction is discussed and exemplified.

Most of the examples given so far have only looked at one exposure and one outcome (e.g. type of food eaten vs. risk of gastroenteritis in Chapter 4, HIV status vs. risk of tuberculosis in Chapter 6, or length of relationship vs. risk of chlamydia infection in the previous chapter). In many instances there may be several factors that are potentially associated with risk of disease. There are two possibilities here.

1. We may want to describe the independent contributions to risk of disease from several factors. Risk of infection with measles in a cohort of children could depend on family size, age, vaccination status, type of schooling, etc. Each of these factors could well play an independent role with regard to the number of measles cases in the cohort during one year, and we may want to analyse them all.

2. Alternatively, we may just want to study the risk associated with a single factor. In the measles example, we might be interested in the association between age at vaccination and subsequent risk of measles infection. All of the other variables, such as family size, etc., would then just be potential confounders, and we would want to get rid of their influences in our calculation of an RR or OR.

From the point of view of the statistical analysis, it does not really matter which approach we choose. Statistics just measures the degree of association between any factor and disease, and is quite blind to the issue of causation or confounding. The decision either to regard the different variables as independently important or to regard one as primarily important and the others as confounders rests with the person who is performing the analysis, and also depends on the exact question being asked.

ADJUSTING FOR CONFOUNDING

In many situations one is quite determined to study just one single risk factor for disease, and potential confounding effects from other factors need to be eliminated as far as possible. In Chapter 5 it was mentioned that confounding can be adjusted for in the analysis, if only data on the confounding variable have been collected. The simplest way to grasp this is described below.

Confounding occurs when the two groups which one is comparing are not equal with regard to some other real risk factor for the disease (other than the factor one wants to study). If only the two groups were equal (i.e. same age distribution, same proportion of women, same nutritional status, etc.), there would be no confounding. One way to solve this is to compare *subgroups* in which the subjects have similar values for the confounding variable, instead of making the comparison between the total of the two original groups. The results of these subgroup comparisons are then averaged in a clever fashion to give an overall RR or OR. These subgroups of subjects who have similar values for a confounder are often called *strata,* and the procedure is called *stratification.* The resulting OR or RR is said to be *adjusted,* and by performing a stratified analysis, we have *controlled* for this confounder.

For example, a study wanted to determine whether the seroprevalence of antibody to infection with herpes simplex virus type 2 (HSV-2) was increasing over time in the population. This disease is mainly spread through sexual intercourse, and the seroprevalence has been suggested to be a good marker of sexual behaviour. Previous studies have shown that the risk of having markers for HSV-2 infection increases with the number of sexual partners a person has had in his or her life.

In order to do this, two random samples of pregnant women in Stockholm were tested for antibody, namely one group of 940 women who were pregnant in 1969, and another group of 1000 women who were pregnant in 1989. The seroprevalence in those 2 years was found to be 17% and 33%, respectively. For the purpose of this example, we shall call the prevalence in 1969 the baseline prevalence, and thus make the women who were pregnant in 1969 our comparison group. The risk ratio for being HSV-2 positive in 1989 compared with 1969 would be 0.33/0.17 = 1.9.

Further analysis showed that in both groups of women there was an increase in seroprevalence with age. This should make us stop and ask ourselves whether there is any other possible difference between the two groups, other than the fact that they were pregnant 20 years apart. What happens if the women in one of the groups were older on average? Since age is associated with prevalence, this fact by itself would make the prevalence higher in that group.

In effect, it was found that the mothers-to-be in 1989 were on average 4.4 years older than those in 1969. As in most industrialized countries, women's age at the birth of their first child (and thus also at the birth of subsequent children) has increased in Sweden in recent decades. This is a nice example of confounding, since the two groups of women differed not only in the year of their pregnancy (which is the factor we wish to study), but also in that the risk factor 'age' was not equally distributed between the two groups.

The way to control for age is to divide the women from both years into strata, where each stratum only contains women from a certain age group. The first stratum consists of the women from 1969 who were aged 25 years or younger at the time of pregnancy, and of the women from 1989 who were also aged 25 years or younger at the time of their pregnancies. The second stratum contains the women aged 26–30 years from both groups, and so on. The relative risk of infection in the women from 1989 is then calculated within each stratum only (i.e. only for women of approximately the same age) (see Table 9.1).

Table 9.1 Prevalence of antibody to herpes simplex virus type 2 by age group in samples of women in Stockholm who were pregnant in 1969 and 1989. The relative risks (RRs) for infection in 1989 are calculated setting the risk in 1969 to 1 for each age group

Age group (years)	1969			1989			RR
	Sero-positive	Number tested	Positive (%)	Sero-positive	Number tested	Positive (%)	
≤25	97	584	16.6	81	255	31.8	1.92
26–30	44	252	17.5	106	352	30.1	1.72
31–35	16	78	20.5	101	259	39.0	1.90
≥36	6	26	23.1	42	134	31.3	1.35
Total	163	940	17.3	330	1000	33.0	1.91

For each age group, the RR is calculated by dividing the seroprevalence in 1989 by the seroprevalence in 1969. You can see that in all but the youngest age groups ('strata'), the RR is lower than the overall RR in the bottom row. If you look closely at the number tested in each age group, you can also see the reason for this. The average age of the women in 1989 was higher – for example, there were 134 women out of 1000 over 35 years of age in 1989 vs. only 26 out of 940 in 1969. Since prevalence was found to increase with age, this difference in age distribution will itself lead to a higher average prevalence in the women of 1989.

If we want one single figure to describe the increased risk of being HSV-2 positive in 1989, we need to adjust for this age difference. One way of doing this would be just to average the RRs for the four age groups. However, the total numbers of women in the four age groups are rather different. Referring back to the discussion about confidence intervals for proportions in Chapter 7, one would be more confident about the figure for seroprevalence in the women aged 25 years or younger in 1969, which is calculated as 97 positive out of 584 tested, than about the figure for women aged over 35 years in 1969, which was based on only 26 women, six of whom were positive.

This intuition is supported by calculating the confidence intervals for each of the RRs. We again use the following formula:

$$\text{error factor} = \exp^{2 \times \sqrt{1/a + 1/b}}$$

where a is the number of positive women in 1969 and b is the number of positive women in 1989. Each RR is then divided and multiplied by its error factor to obtain an upper and lower limit. (You will notice that for the last RR this is not quite permitted, since one really needs at least 10 cases in each group, but we shall disregard this here.)

The corresponding confidence intervals are listed in Table 9.2. It is evident that the group with the lowest number of cases has the widest confidence interval.

Table 9.2 Confidence intervals for the relative risks (RR) for the study in Table 9.1

Age group (years)	RR	95% Confidence interval
≤25	1.92	1.50–2.71
26–30	1.72	1.20–2.46
31–35	1.90	1.11–3.25
≥36	1.35	0.56–3.23

The following description of Mantel–Haenszel weighted ratios is rather technical, and you might be satisfied just to know that an adjusted risk ratio can be calculated. However, I shall include this information anyway for future reference, and should you ever want to calculate an adjusted RR or OR, the text below will show you how to do it.

If one wants to average the four values for relative risks in the above herpes example properly, one should not take the plain average of the four numbers, but rather give them different weights depending on how reliable each of the four RRs is. In this context 'reliable' is taken to mean the same as 'having a narrow confidence interval'. The narrower the confidence interval, the more credible is the RR, and the higher the weight it gets. The best way to do this is to use a scheme described by Mantel and Haenszel, where each subgroup RR is given a weight in the following way.

1. Take the number of cases in the baseline or *unexposed* group (women pregnant in 1969 in this case). If we use the 26–30 years age group as an example, this number would be 44.

2. Multiply by the total number of individuals in the *exposed* group (which here would be the women pregnant in 1989). There were 352 women in the 26–30 years age group in 1989.

3. Divide by the total number of individuals in that age group, adding the 1969 and 1989 women. This would be $252 + 352 = 604$ for the 26–30 years age group.

4. The resulting figure is the Mantel–Haenszel weight of the RR for women in that age group: $44 \times 352/(252 + 352) = 25.6$.

   For all of the age groups, the Mantel–Haenszel weights would be as follows:

   $\leqslant 25$: $\qquad w_{\leqslant 25} = 97 \times \dfrac{255}{584 + 255} = 29.5$

   26–30: $\qquad w_{26-30} = 44 \times \dfrac{352}{252 + 352} = 25.6$

   31–35: $\qquad w_{31-35} = 16 \times \dfrac{259}{78 + 259} = 12.3$

   $36 \geqslant$: $\qquad w_{36\geqslant} = 6 \times \dfrac{134}{26 + 134} = 5.0$

where w denotes 'weight'. We can see that the weight is highest for the group for which we have most data, and lowest where the number of women (and seropositive women) is lowest.

5. Each of the RRs is then multiplied by its corresponding weight and the four products are added.

6. This number is divided by the sum of all the weights. The final resulting number is the Mantel–Haenszel estimate of the adjusted RR:

$$RR_{MH} = \frac{(1.92 \times 29.5) + (1.72 \times 25.6) + (1.90 \times 12.3) + (1.35 \times 5.0)}{29.5 + 25.6 + 12.3 + 5.0} = 1.82$$

This adjustment procedure has thus lowered the estimated RR from a *crude* value for the overall total of 1.91 in the table above to an *adjusted* value of 1.82. What we have done is to recognize that the women who were pregnant in 1989 were older on average, and by calculating an RR_{MH} we have effectively erased the effect of this confounder.

A point should be made about words here. 'Adjusted' sounds impressive, and one immediately senses that an adjusted RR must be much better than a crude one – perhaps it is even the 'true' RR. Just remember, once again, that we can only adjust for the confounders of which we are aware, and for which we have data. If unknown confounders of the study exist that have not been taken into account, no elaborate Mantel–Haenszel weighting scheme will be able to adjust for them. 'Adjusted' means adjusted for the confounders that we were able to imagine and measure, and nothing else.

This was an example of a cross-sectional study, in which risks and RRs could be calculated. If we are trying to adjust an OR from a case–control study for confounding, this can be done in exactly the same way, by calculating an OR for each stratum. The weights for these ORs are then calculated in the same way, but points 1 to 3 above would instead read as follows.

Make a separate 2×2 table for each stratum. Then for each table:

1. take the number of unexposed cases (if you look back at the general 2×2 table of Chapter 5, this would correspond to c);

2. multiply by the number of exposed controls (b in the general 2×2 table);

3. divide by the total number of individuals in that stratum ($= a + b + c + d$).

This gives you the weight of the OR for this stratum, and they are then added as in points 5 and 6 above to give an adjusted OR_{MH}.

In our study of pregnant women, it does seem that there had been a real increase in HSV-2 seroprevalence between 1969 and 1989, since the adjusted RR was 1.82. This could indicate that the second group of women had had a higher number of partners on average before the blood sample was taken in connection with a pregnancy. In non-infectious disease epidemiology, this would have been the obvious explanation – the women from 1989 had had almost twice as many sexual partners as the women from 1969. But remember that we are dealing with infections here. If the prevalence of HSV-2 infection had increased in men during the 20-year period, then the risk of becoming infected by any single partner would have increased. In reality, what had probably happened is that an initial increase in prevalence in one of the sexes led to a higher risk of infection per partner for the other sex. This in turn would lead to the first sex being more exposed per partner, and so on in an upward spiral. Thus the 80% increase in prevalence is surely not explained by an almost doubling of the number of sexual partners, but by a mixture of more partners and an increased risk per partner in a way that is difficult to elucidate precisely.

One more point should be made about confounding. A confounder is not something that is inherent to the data one is perusing. As was pointed out in Chapter 5, it is also a question of perspective. In the above example, we wanted to use seroprevalence of antibody to HSV-2 as a measure of changes in sexual behaviour between 1969 and 1989, which meant that we had to adjust for the age difference. Another aspect of HSV-2 infection is that it can be transmitted from mother to child during delivery and cause a serious disease in the newborn. An equally important question could therefore have been: 'What was the risk for a baby being born in 1989 compared with one being born in 1969 of having a mother who was seropositive for HSV-2?'. The answer to this question would be the crude risk ratio of 1.91, since the average risk to all babies would have nothing to do with the mothers' age distribution in the different years.

MATCHING

There is another rather obvious way to control for possible confounders at the stage of data collection, and that is to match the controls to the cases. Confounding arises when there is an imbalance between the groups with regard to some risk factor for disease other than the one we want to study. Put another way, when comparing a certain outcome (e.g. attack rate) in two different groups, we want them to be as similar as possible in all respects, except for the factor that we wish to study (e.g. vaccination status). One way to achieve this in a case–control study is to select controls that are similar to the cases with regard to all of the suspected confounders, such as age, sex, family size, school attended, etc. If we succeed in this, we will have controlled for these confounders in the study proper, and need not concern ourselves with the stratification methods described above, or the regression methods described below.

The analysis of a matched study becomes slightly different to that of a non-matched study. We shall not compare all of the cases to all of the controls, but rather analyse the differences within each matched pair. Let us look at an artificial example. Suppose that we decide we want to study the association between 'being a health-care worker' and 'having markers of hepatitis B infection'. We could then select a group of health-care workers, choose a control for each person of the same sex and age, and test the members of each pair for hepatitis B markers.

The result could be presented in a slightly modified 2×2 table such as the one below:

		Control:		
		Positive for markers	Negative for markers	
Health-care worker:	Positive for markers	10	30	40
	Negative for markers	20	90	110
		30	120	150

This table shows that we have studied 150 pairs (150 health-care workers matched to 150 controls). In 100 of these pairs, both subjects had the same hepatitis B status – in 10 pairs both were positive, and in 90 pairs both were negative. These pairs add nothing to our analysis, and are disregarded.

The interesting cells are the upper right-hand and lower left-hand ones, in which the pairs are *discordant* with regard to hepatitis B status. If there was no extra risk of being positive if one was a health-care worker, we would expect the numbers in these two cells to be about the same, disregarding randomly introduced differences from sampling.

If we want to test for the statistical significance of the outcome in a matched study, we use something called McNemar's χ^2 test. If we call the number of pairs in the upper right-hand cell b and the number of pairs in the lower left-hand cell c, then the test value becomes:

$$\chi^2 = \frac{(|b - c| - 1)^2}{b + c} \quad (1 \text{ df})$$

where the straight lines on either side of $|b - c|$ mean that we should take the absolute value of the difference (i.e. disregard the minus sign if there is one). In our example about hepatitis B, the value would be as follows:

$$\chi^2 = \frac{(|30 - 20| - 1)^2}{30 + 20} = \frac{81}{50} = 1.62$$

The χ^2 value for McNemar's test has 1 degree of freedom, which means that it has to be greater than 3.84 for our finding to be significant at the 5% level. We conclude that in this matched study the slight difference in sero-prevalence between the groups could easily be just a chance finding.

Just as in the cautionary note about adjusting in the previous section, it is important to realize that matching only takes care of these potential additional factors that were the basis for the matching. There may well be other confounders involved that we are either unaware of or cannot match for, and these could still distort the result of a study. In fact, one disadvantage of matched studies is that it becomes difficult to control for other confounders in the analysis.

In general, the introduction of matching in a study requires more work, since many of the potential controls will have to be discarded due to lack of a matching case. In many situations it becomes simpler to control for confounders in the statistical analysis than to do extensive work trying to find matching controls.

REGRESSION MODELS

Nowadays, most epidemiological studies are analysed with some type of regression model. A number of computer programs exist for this purpose, with varying degrees of sophistication, including the very powerful packages SAS, GLIM and SPSS, which require considerable knowledge of computing and statistics, and the more immediately accessible EGRET, EpiInfo, STATA and JMP.

Regression models are often called 'linear models' or 'multiple regression models'. For the calculation of ORs and RRs one often uses a variant called 'logistic regression models'.

The basic idea in all regression is to fit a line to a number of data points in a diagram. In Figure 9.1 we assume that we have tested for antibody to some disease in 110 children aged 5 to 15 years, 10 children from each year group.

The degree to which such a line fits the data is in principle measured by considering the vertical distances of each point from the line. If all of the points are quite close to the line this is regarded as a good fit, whereas large distances indicate that the regression line does not describe the data very well.

In epidemiology the question is usually about the effects of exposure. In the above example we would ask whether there is any statistical indication

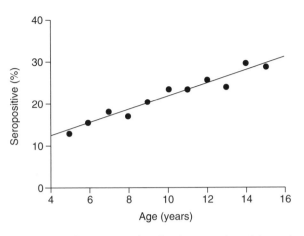

Figure 9.1   An example of a regression line fitted to a number of data points.

that seropositivity increases with age, or whether we obtained the curve just by chance. If there really was no increase with age, we would assume that the best estimate of seroprevalence in this group would be the overall average, which in this case can be calculated to be 21% for all 110 children. This would also be the expected figure for each age class, and in this case the curve would be as shown in Figure 9.2.

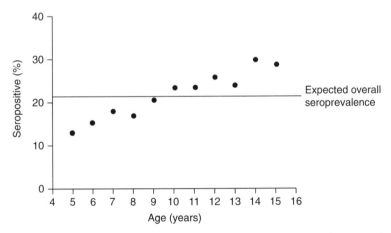

Figure 9.2   Some data points as in Figure 9.1, now with a line showing the expected seroprevalence if there were no association between age and seropositivity.

The statistical analysis then consists of comparing how this last *model*, in which seroprevalence is assumed not to vary with age, fits the data, compared with the model with the sloping line above. The strength of the evidence for the slope model depends partly on the steepness of the slope and partly on the amount of variation around the average value of each year group. In this example it seems rather obvious that there is an increase with age.

Even a simple 2 × 2 table could be analysed like this, but then we would no longer have numerical values along the horizontal axis. Instead there will be two *categories*, as in the following example measuring the protective effect of a hypothetical vaccine in a case–control study:

	Ill	Healthy	
Vaccinated	20	75	95
Not vaccinated	80	25	105
	100	100	200

The odds of being vaccinated ('being exposed to the factor vaccination') will be 20/80 = 0.25 in the group of cases, compared with 75/25 = 3 in the group of controls. The OR for having been vaccinated if one did not fall ill in this example would be 3/0.25 = 12, and its statistical significance could be tested by calculating the confidence interval as described in Chapter 5.

A similar calculation could be performed with a regression model. The advantage of this method will not be immediately evident from this simple example, but will be explained below. For reasons of calculation, one often converts the odds into their logarithms when using a regression method, which explains the name 'logistic regression'. The natural logarithms of the odds above are

$$\ln(0.25) = -1.39$$
$$\ln(3) = 1.10$$

and these two values are illustrated as shown in Figure 9.3.

The overall odds of being vaccinated among all 200 subjects was 95/105 = 0.90, with the corresponding logarithm $\ln(0.90) = -0.11$. If the vaccine was completely ineffective, and there was no association between vaccination and risk of disease, the expected ln(odds) for both categories would thus have been −0.11.

We could now imagine drawing a regression line through the two points, and comparing it with a horizontal line through ln(odds) = −0.11, just as we

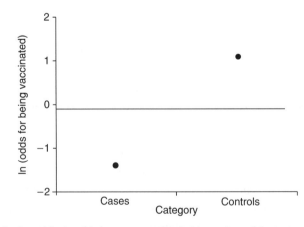

Figure 9.3 Logarithmic odds for exposure (i.e. being vaccinated) in cases and controls. The solid line through ln(odds) = −0.11 corresponds to the value for the whole group (no difference between cases and controls).

did in Figure 9.2 above. A logistic regression programme will give an estimate for the slope and also a statistical significance value (i.e. the probability that the observed slope would occur just by chance even if the true slope was in reality zero – that is the horizontal line). If the case category is given the value $x = 0$ and the control category $x = 1$, then the slope would be $(1.10 - [-1.39])/1 = 2.49$. Since subtracting two logarithms amounts to the same thing as taking the logarithm of the quotient, or

$$\ln(a) - \ln(b) = \ln(a/b)$$

this must mean that 2.49 is the logarithm of the two odds divided. However, the quotient of the two odds is the definition of the odds ratio, and thus

$$1.10 - (-1.39) = \ln(3/0.25) = 2.49 = \ln(OR).$$

If $\ln(OR) = 2.49$, exponentiation of both sides gives the following:

$$\exp^{\ln(OR)} = OR = \exp^{2.49} = 12$$

which is the same as the odds ratio calculated from the table.

This may seem a very roundabout way of doing a simple calculation. The strength of regression methods comes from the fact that they directly control for confounders. If we want to study the effect of a vaccine as in the above example, we may have to take into account other differences between the two categories in the table. There may be different age distributions in the two groups (e.g. the unvaccinated individuals being younger). There may be social differences (e.g. the unvaccinated individuals coming from poorer backgrounds with larger families, which would mean that they were possibly more exposed), and so on. Let us say that we could divide the children into those younger or older than 1 year, and into three social classes. In order to control for confounding with non-regression methods we would then have to construct six 2×2 tables like the one above, one for each possible combination of age and social class, thus making a stratified analysis as shown overleaf.

We could then calculate an overall odds ratio for being vaccinated in cases vs. controls according to the Mantel–Haenszel procedure described above. This is clearly quite a laborious task, and there might also be some combinations of age and social class for which there were very few subjects in the table, making estimates unreliable.

All of this work becomes unnecessary when using a computer program for logistic regression. One just enters all of the subjects, together with their vaccination status, age, social class and outcome. The program then fits the best possible linear combination to the data, and the OR for vaccination status given by the program will be adjusted for the other two variables.

(For the mathematically inclined, it might be pointed out that the program fits a hyperplane in n space through all of the data points, where $n - 1$ is the number of input variables, and the last axis is the outcome variable. This is

Age less than 1 year

Social class 1

	III	Healthy
Vaccinated	X	X
Unvaccinated	X	X

Social class 2

	III	Healthy
Vaccinated	X	X
Unvaccinated	X	X

Social class 3

	III	Healthy
Vaccinated	X	X
Unvaccinated	X	X

Age greater than 1 year

Social class 1

	III	Healthy
Vaccinated	X	X
Unvaccinated	X	X

Social class 2

	III	Healthy
Vaccinated	X	X
Unvaccinated	X	X

Social class 3

	III	Healthy
Vaccinated	X	X
Unvaccinated	X	X

most easily visualized for a study with two variables – for example, vaccination status along the x-axis, age along the y-axis, and outcome along the z-axis. Each subject will be a point in this space, and the algorithm will fit the best plane through all of these points. The intersection of this plane with the x-z-plane will be the regression line for outcome vs. vaccination status, controlled for age, and the intersection with the y-z-plane will show the outcome for different ages, controlled for vaccination status (a regression program does not differentiate between the variables under study and the confounders; it regards all variables as equal). Incidentally, if you read articles in which regression has been used in the analysis, you may come across the term *covariate*. This word is a favourite with statisticians, and it means the same as 'variable' or 'factor' (i.e. any of the exposures entered into the regression model to be tested against the outcome). In this example, vaccination status and age would be the two covariates analysed.)

Regression programs are thus very powerful and efficient. However, there is one great danger in entering all of the data into such a program and pressing the 'go' button. The algorithm is essentially a 'black box', and as soon as more than a few variables are included for each subject, it becomes impossible to perceive how the fitting is actually done. Therefore it is always good epidemiological practice to start the analysis with some simple graphs, and some 2×2 tables using rough divisions of the variables, just to get some feel for the data. It is also good practice to let the regression program analyse the variables under study and the confounders one at a time before they are entered jointly in the model. This strategy is called 'univariate analysis', and it usually reveals the most important associations and the strongest confounders. Any major change between an OR or an RR for an exposure given in the univariate analysis and the corresponding adjusted OR or RR should always be investigated. It could be due to strong confounding from another variable, but it could also be due to some erroneous assumptions in the model. One such additional problem is called *interaction*, and this will be the subject of the next section.

INTERACTION

It is not easy to grasp immediately the assumptions that are usually made when risk of disease is analysed for several variables simultaneously, either by stratified analysis or by regression models.

One such standard assumption is that risks are added in a multiplicative fashion. Suppose that our study shows that individuals with risk factor A have twice the risk of disease (adjusted for confounders) compared with those who do not have risk factor A. We have also found that individuals with risk factor B have a three times higher risk than those without it (still adjusted for confounders). Stratified analysis as well as regression models then postulate that a person who has both A *and* B as risk factors will be at $2 \times 3 = 6$ times higher risk of disease than a person who has neither of these risk factors. Whereas this may be true for a number of exposures and diseases, one really needs a knowledge of the actual mechanisms to be able to judge whether this assumption is correct. For example, studies have shown that alcoholism and lack of an increase in white blood cell count on arrival at hospital are both risk factors for dying from acute pneumococcal pneumonia. It is not self-evident that a patient with both of these risk factors would have the multiplied risk of dying, since one feels that the way in which the factors interplay should be important. Nevertheless, multiplicative risk is implicitly assumed in most epidemiological analyses, and this fact should be questioned more than it usually is.

Another standard assumption is that a true OR or RR for disease from a certain exposure does exist, and that this is independent of the actual values of other variables. This true value might be distorted by confounders, but if the latter are adjusted for properly, we should obtain a single, dependable value. In a stratified analysis such as the one for vaccine efficacy with the six 2×2 tables above, the OR for disease according to vaccination status should be the same in each of the six tables. There may be statistical variations between the ORs of the different tables due to sampling, but this is being handled by the Mantel–Haenszel analysis, which gives the best estimate of an overall value from all six tables.

However, there may well be situations in which the actual value of an OR or RR varies with different values for other variables. An example of such interaction comes from a study in Brazil, where risk factors for children dying from an infection were analysed in a case–control study[1]. The main objective was to investigate whether breastfeeding protected against infant deaths from infectious diseases.

During 1985, data were collected on all infant (less than 1 year of age) deaths from infectious causes in an area of southern Brazil. For each case, two infants in the immediate neighbourhood were chosen as controls. The mothers were interviewed about feeding practices, and also about a large number of possible confounders, such as birth order, birth weight, income, water source, antenatal care, mode of delivery, etc. Adjusted ORs for dying from an infection for those children who were only given milk other than mother's milk were compared with those who were exclusively breastfed (see Table 9.3).

Table 9.3 Odds ratios (OR) for dying from infectious causes in non-breastfed compared to breastfed children in a study from Brazil (*Source*: Victora et al.[1])

	OR
Diarrhoea	14.2
Respiratory infection	3.6
Other infection	2.5

However, if the ORs were calculated separately for infants aged less than 2 months and infants aged 2 to 11 months, the results change (see Table 9.4).

For respiratory and other infections, the influence of feeding practices on the risk of death does not seem to differ much with age. However, for

Table 9.4 The same odds ratios as in Table 9.3, now broken down by age group

	Age group	
	< 2 months	2–11 months
Diarrhoea	23.3	5.3
Respiratory infection	4.1	3.4
Other infection	1.9	2.0

diarrhoeal deaths there is a huge difference in the evident protection given by breastfeeding.

It is interesting to speculate about this difference in risks, and whether the protection is due to anti-infective properties of breast milk, or perhaps to the fact that a breastfed infant will not come into contact with sources of water that may be contaminated. Which of these mechanisms would be most likely to explain the difference in risk with age? We shall evade these questions here, and instead concentrate on the methodological implications of the finding.

How should one give an overall OR for the association between the factor 'not breastfeeding' and death from diarrhoea in this study? The answer is that it should probably not be done. Thus the question 'To what extent does breastfeeding protect young children from diarrhoea?' does not have a simple numerical answer. The answer is 'That depends on the age of the child'. The OR assumes different values in the two different age groups, and to give one value would be misleading in that it would conceal an important interaction between this risk factor and age. Table 9.4 above tells us something about our study subjects, and this information should not be discarded by just giving an overall OR.

Another example of interaction comes from the study of risk factors for chlamydia infection mentioned in Chapter 8[2]. Around 6000 young women were interviewed about their sexual lifestyle and tested for asymptomatic chlamydia infection. One of the questions was 'Have you had any sexually transmitted disease before?'. In a univariate analysis (i.e. just comparing the prevalence in those who had not previously had any STI with the prevalence in those who had), it was found that previous infection was associated with a slightly lower risk of being chlamydia positive in the study (OR = 0.77). When the answers to this question were stratified according to the age of the women, the odds for being chlamydia infected in the three age groups emerged as shown in Table 9.5.

This table shows that in this group of women, reported previous STI was a strong risk factor for present chlamydia infection among the youngest subjects, whereas in the two older groups there almost seemed to be a protective effect from previous STIs. In this example the interaction is even more evident than in the example about diarrhoea, since it tends to work in opposite directions in the different strata.

Table 9.5 Interaction between the risk factor 'previous sexually transmitted infection (STI)' and age in a study on chlamydia infection in Sweden (*Source:* Ramstedt et al.[2])

Age group (years)	Previous STI	No previous STI	OR
17	3.95	1.00	3.95/1.00 = 3.95
18–23	1.95	2.74	1.95/2.74 = 0.71
24	1.44	1.95	1.44/1.95 = 0.74

These are two real-life examples of interaction between two variables in an analysis where the OR for one is not independent of the value for the other. When making a stratified analysis like the one described above, one should always check whether the ORs for the various strata seem to be very different, as this could indicate interaction. In no analysis will the ORs be exactly the same for all strata (look at the example concerning herpes infection in pregnant women in Table 9.1), and the problem is to decide whether the variation in ORs is a mere statistical fluctuation around one true value, or whether there is evidence of interaction. Statistical tests for this problem do exist, but they are not very powerful, and the decision remains largely one of common sense.

Computer programs for linear regression usually allow the possibility of entering interaction variables in the analysis. This is done by indicating which two variables should interact, and then running the model again to see whether this improves the regression fit significantly compared with a model with no interaction. Some of the more advanced programs have built-in algorithms that decide when interaction occurs, but even those do not totally alleviate the necessity for common sense and experience in judging whether the assumed interaction is justified by the increase in fit.

Another interaction that is sometimes used in epidemiological literature is *effect modification,* which neatly summarizes the concept of the effect of some exposure being modified by the value of another variable. One practical problem that arises when interaction appears in a study is that the concept may be quite difficult to explain to people with little experience in epidemiology. Tables will become more messy, and it may be impossible to answer straightforward questions about the magnitude of a certain risk.

MISCLASSIFICATION

There is one additional risk with logistic regression models, and that concerns the precision with which we are able to measure the variables analysed. If data on one real risk factor can only be assessed rather crudely, with a high degree of misclassification of individuals, whereas data on a confounder can be measured very precisely, then the regression may show a significant independent influence of risk of disease from the confounder[3]. An example comes from studies of cervical cancer, where one risk factor analysed has been previous STIs and another has been smoking. If the probability of previous STIs is assessed as 'number of past sexual partners', this becomes a very crude measure, since the real risk was whether or not any of those partners were infectious with an STI. Many women will be misclassified by this measure. Smoking, on the other hand, can be assessed rather precisely. The result of such an analysis could be (and has been) that after controlling for the number of partners, smoking still remains an independent risk factor.

Although this may be a true association, it could also be explained by our inability to measure the risk of previous STI correctly.

SUMMARY

In many situations one wishes to analyse the association between several different factors (age, sex, vaccination status, family size, time of year, nutritional status, etc.) and the risk of disease. Epidemiological studies will often collect data on a number of potential risk factors, and the analysis should include those factors that are thought to be either causally related to the disease or possibly subject to confounding.

Confounding can be controlled by stratification, where the two groups one wishes to compare are divided into subgroups, each subgroup consisting of only the subjects who have similar values for the confounder. A comparison is then made by comparing not the two original large groups, but only the pairs of subgroups with similar values for the confounder. From each pairwise comparison a value is obtained for an OR or an RR, and these values can then be averaged by the Mantel–Haenszel algorithm to give an adjusted value that is applicable to the original group comparison.

Matching is another way of controlling for confounding, whereby from the beginning a control is chosen for each case that has similar values for the confounder. The analysis of matched studies becomes slightly different.

Most reasonably large data sets are now analysed by some type of regression method. The advantage of these methods is that they can control for several different confounders simultaneously, and also reveal several independent risk factors. Their main drawback is that the analysis becomes opaque, and one loses the feel for what is really happening with the data.

If the association between a risk factor and an outcome is influenced by the value of some other risk factor, these two risk factors are said to interact.

REFERENCES

1. Victora CG, Vaughan JP, Lombardi C *et al.* Evidence for protection by breast-feeding against infant deaths from infectious diseases in Brazil. *Lancet* 1987; **2**: 319–22.
2. Ramstedt K, Forssman L, Giesecke J, Granath F. Risk factors for *Chlamydia trachomatis* infection in 6810 young women attending family planning clinics. *Int J STD AIDS* 1992; **3**: 117–22.
3. Phillips AN, Davey Smith G. How independent are 'independent' effects? Relative risk estimation when correlated exposures are measured imprecisely. *J Clin Epidemiol* 1991; **44**: 1223–31.

Chapter 10
Survival analysis

Here we deal with the study of time periods until something happens, such as incubation times, recovery times, etc. An example of how to perform a survival analysis is presented, and the difference between risks and rates is discussed.

Often in epidemiology we are only interested in whether or not something happened, but not exactly when. For example, we may want to know *if* someone was infected or not in order to be able to calculate an attack rate, or we may want to know *if* a patient with gastroenteritis ate a specific food item or not in order to calculate an odds ratio. In both of these examples it does not matter very much exactly when these events took place. However, in infectious disease epidemiology we are also quite often interested in *when* something occurred. Examples of such questions are calculation of incubation times, or the proportion of a population that was infected at a given date during an epidemic. We shall look more closely at these issues later in this book, but this section introduces the theoretical background to such analyses.

SURVIVAL ANALYSIS

When one wants to study time periods until something happens, one always starts with a cohort of individuals who are followed over time, much as in the example of rates and person-years given in Chapter 6. For example, we may want to study the time to death in people who develop cirrhosis from chronic active hepatitis (this is an example of the type of study that has given this method its name: how many people survive for 1, 2, 3, etc. years after developing cirrhosis?). Another example concerns the problem of waning immunity after vaccination. In the absence of natural boosters, how long will it be before we start to see cases among people who were immunized as children? In this example, 'survival' will denote the proportion of people who still have not contracted the disease 20, 30, 50, etc. years after vaccination.

If the time periods we are trying to measure are short, like the average incubation time in an outbreak of food poisoning, there is really no need to get into survival analysis. However, if the time periods we are looking at are long or very long, there may be at least three problems with such studies.

1. The outcome we are looking for may not have happened to all of the people in the cohort. Cohort studies are often lengthy and expensive, and

it may not be feasible to continue the project until everyone has developed the disease, or died, etc.

2. We may lose contact with some of the subjects of the study before it has finished, and so do not know what happened to them. In most practical situations this becomes more of a problem the longer a study runs. These patients are called 'losses to follow-up', and they always create difficulties in cohort studies. In the above example of death from cirrhosis, we cannot just disregard people who were lost to follow-up as if they had never been in the cohort, since one reason for losing contact with them may be that they have died from cirrhosis. If such patients were selectively deleted from our cohort, we would underestimate the risk of death in the cohort. It might also be the other way around – that some people felt so healthy that they stopped coming to the clinic for follow-ups. If those patients were discarded we would overestimate the risk of death in the cohort.

    However, if many of the subjects who were losses to follow-up remained in the cohort for a long time and we knew that they had not developed the outcome when we lost contact with them, then this fact should contain some information, and it would seem uneconomical not to make use of it.

3. Some people in the cohort may suddenly be unable to develop the outcome. For example, if we are studying death from cirrhosis, then patients who die from other causes cannot take part in the study any longer. If we are studying the incidence of hepatitis B infection in a cohort of injecting drug users and one of the subjects is then vaccinated in another clinic, he can no longer give any information to our study.

As you can see, all of the above three points really only relate to problems of cohort studies that are extended in time, but then again, such studies are becoming more and more common even in infectious disease epidemiology.

TERMINOLOGY

The term 'survival analysis' comes from the original application of this method to demographic data, as when one wants to calculate average life expectancy in a population. However, the outcome we are studying does not have to be death. It could be 'becoming infected', or even something positive such as 'recovering from an infection' (e.g. hepatitis B carriers becoming antigen negative). We shall call the outcome we are studying the *event*, where the event could be something either negative or positive to the patient.

Some subjects in our cohort will experience the event, and we can measure the time from the start of the study until this happens for each one of them. However, this will not happen to the subjects in the three groups described above (or at least we shall never know about it for those who are lost to follow-up). These subjects are *censored*, and that could happen for any of the three reasons listed above, namely:

1. the subject had not experienced the event when the study finished;

2. the subject was lost to follow-up from a specified date;

3. the subject experienced an excluding event on a specified date.

For all subjects, whether they were censored or not, we shall at least know the length of time that they spent in the cohort. In most clinical studies, the times will be counted as scheduled visits, and if the event is not directly observable by the patient (e.g. losing hepatitis B surface antigen), it will usually be assumed to have happened on the date of the first visit it was recorded. If the time between visits is long, one sometimes sets the midpoint between the last visit when the event was not observed and the first visit at which it was, to be the time of the event. In a similar manner, losses to follow-up should be included only up to the last visit they attended, not to the first one they missed.

AN ILLUSTRATIVE EXAMPLE

Suppose that we want to answer the following question. How long does an injection of gamma-globulin give protection against infection with hepatitis A in an endemic area?

The simplest way to answer this question would be to give gamma-globulin to a large group of people who had not had hepatitis A, send them away to a country where the virus was common, keep them under observation there for a long period, and then record when the cases started to appear. This would be a regular cohort study.

In reality, this would be difficult to achieve, even though studies like these have actually been performed on Western military personnel stationed in tropical countries. A more everyday situation would be that individuals came to the study country at different times, and stayed there for differing lengths of time. Suppose we chose to study 12 subjects (which is of course far too small a number to achieve any statistical significance, but it will suffice for this example) who we knew would be travelling to the endemic country at any time between January this year and March next year. They were given gamma-globulin just before they left home. Table 10.1 shows the collected data.

In Figure 10.1 these data are displayed in a graph, with months along the *x*-axis and each person as a line, just as in Chapter 6 (see Figure 6.1). The infections (i.e. events) are marked by a short vertical line at the end of the corresponding line.

Table 10.1 Example of input data for a survival analysis. A total of 12 subjects were given gamma-globulin just before they departed to a hepatitis A endemic area, and were subsequently followed for varying lengths of time

Subject	Month departed	Month diagnosed	Comment
1	February	November	—
2	September	—	Still abroad, healthy
3	March	—	Returned home in August, healthy
4	January	—	Lost contact in March
5	January	—	Still abroad, healthy
6	October	—	Returned home in January of second year, healthy
7	June	—	Received new dose of gamma-globulin in July
8	April	August	—
9	March	—	Returned home in April, healthy
10	August	—	Lost contact in January of second year
11	July	January of second year	—
12	January of second year	—	Still abroad, healthy

Subjects 1, 8 and 11 experienced the event (i.e. they had hepatitis A), but all of the others are censored for the following reasons:

- subjects 2, 5 and 12 because they had not experienced the event at the end of the study period;

- subjects 4 and 10 because they were lost to follow-up;

- subjects 3, 6 and 9 because they were no longer exposed; and

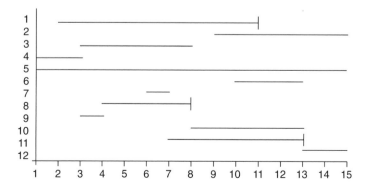

Figure 10.1 Line diagram representing 12 people given gamma-globulin. A short vertical bar indicates an event, in this case the diagnosis of a hepatitis A infection.

- subject 7 because he received a new dose of gamma-globulin, which invalidated the experiment.

The graph looks rather messy. One obvious thing to do, since we are not interested in exact dates but rather in time spent in the cohort, would be to imagine that everyone had the same time of entry, namely the day on which they were injected. This would correspond to pulling all the lines in the graph to the left border. At the same time, we rearrange the order of the subjects according to length of stay (see Figure 10.2).

We can see that no case appears before 4 months of stay, but that after that time, people start contracting hepatitis A infections. One person stays for 14 months without becoming infected. We could rearrange Table 10.1 in the same way, letting 'I' denote infected and 'C' denote censored, where we no longer differentiate between the reasons for censoring (see Table 10.2).

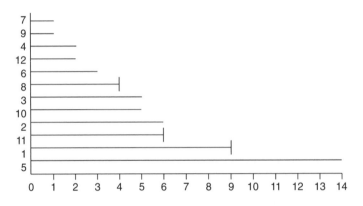

Figure 10.2   The same group of people as in Figure 10.1, but this time ordered according to length of follow-up in the study.

Table 10.2 Data for the same subjects as in Table 10.1, now arranged according to follow-up time (C denotes censored and I denotes infected)

Subject	Months in study	Outcome
7	1	C
9	1	C
4	2	C
12	2	C
6	3	C
8	4	I
3	5	C
10	5	C
2	6	C
11	6	I
1	9	I
5	14	C

The survival curve that we want to construct would show the chance of remaining uninfected after a certain number of months in the cohort (or conversely the risk of having become infected after a certain number of months). The way to calculate this is to draw up a new table as follows.

1. List all of the months according to the above table, using months in the cohort for each subject, not the actual calendar month of the events.

2. In the second column, list how many individuals were left in the cohort at the beginning of that month. Call that number n_i, where n_1 is the number in the first row, n_2 is the number in the second row, and so on.

3. In the third column, list how many events (infections in this case) occurred during that month. Call that number I_i, where I_1 is the first row, I_2 is the second row, etc. For several of the months, I_i will just be zero.

4. In the fourth column list how many people (if any) were censored during that month.

In our example, the table thus far would look like Table 10.3.

Table 10.3 The first steps in the construction of a table for a survival analysis

Month	n_i	I_i	Censored
1	12	0	2
2	10	0	2
3	8	0	1
4	7	1	0
5	6	0	2
6	4	1	1
7	2	0	0
8	2	0	0
9	2	1	0
10	1	0	0
11	1	0	0
12	1	0	0
13	1	0	0
14	1	0	1

This table should read as follows. In the first line, we can see that 12 people entered the cohort. Two of these individuals were censored during the first month. The second line thus shows that 10 people remained in the cohort at the beginning of the second month, and that two of these were censored during that month. The first event appeared in month 4, line 4. You can see that each n_i is equal to the n_i in the line above minus the events and censorings in that line.

At the beginning of each month there is obviously a number n_i, who could fall ill during that month. In some of the months one of the subjects is diagnosed with hepatitis infection, and in some not. The best estimate of the risk of becoming a case during month i is the number of cases during that month divided by the number of subjects at its beginning, or I/n_i. The probability of not becoming a case during month i is obviously the converse. That is, $n_i - I_i$ subjects out of the total n_i did not become infected, and the 'risk of not becoming infected' will thus be $(n_i - I_i)/n_i = 1 - I_i/n_i$. Any subject who was still healthy at the beginning of month i would have the chance $(1 - I_i/n_i)$ of remaining healthy at the end of the month.

A basic fact of statistical theory is that the collective chance of A and B and C occurring is the same as the likelihood that A happens multiplied by the likelihood that B happens multiplied by the likelihood that C happens. In our example, this would mean that the chance of remaining healthy after, say, three time periods can be calculated as the likelihood of escaping infection during the first period, multiplied by the likelihood of remaining healthy during the second period, multiplied by the likelihood of not becoming a case during the third period.

This is all rather difficult when described in words like this. It becomes simpler when one uses mathematics.

5. Next, in a fifth column, calculate $1 - I_i/n_i$ for each line. Call this number L_i (where 'L' denotes being lucky and escaping disease). For the months when there are no cases, L_i will just be equal to 1.

6. Finally, call the numbers of the sixth column S_i (where 'S' denotes survival). They are calculated by multiplying S_i in the line above with L_i to the left (i.e. $S_{i+1} = S_i \times L_{i+1}$). For the first line, S_1 is defined as $L_1 \times 1$. Each S_i is an estimate of the chance of still remaining uninfected just at the end of the corresponding month.

Table 10.4 shows the final table.

Figure 10.3 shows how the S_i values are plotted against time to obtain the survival curve (often called the Kaplan–Meier plot, after its inventors).

This curve quite nicely sums up what we want to know. It shows that infections start appearing about 4 months after the injection with gamma-globulin, and that the risk of becoming a case increases rather linearly after that. The median time until diagnosis seems to be about 9 months. (The risk of becoming infected with hepatitis A in this hypothetical country must be very high, and the gamma-globulin seems to wear off faster than in real life, so please do not regard this as a very realistic example.)

The further to the right we move along the survival curve, the fewer subjects will be left on which to base our estimates of L_i and S_i. This means that the latter part of such a curve will always be more uncertain than the first

Table 10.4 The final table for the survival analysis in Table 10.1. S_i is an estimate of the probability of remaining uninfected at the end of month number i

Month	n_i	I_i	Censored	L_i	S_i
1	12	0	2	1	1
2	10	0	2	1	1
3	8	0	1	1	1
4	7	1	0	0.86	0.86
5	6	0	2	1	0.86
6	4	1	1	0.75	0.64
7	2	0	0	1	0.64
8	2	0	0	1	0.64
9	2	1	0	0.5	0.32
10	1	0	0	1	0.32
11	1	0	0	1	0.32
12	1	0	0	1	0.32
13	1	0	0	1	0.32
14	1	0	1	1	0.32

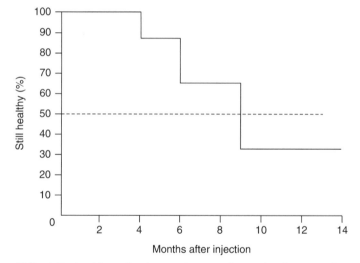

Figure 10.3 A Kaplan–Meier plot showing the survival curve for the data in Table 10.1.

part. It is good practice to indicate the number of subjects still at risk after each event on the curve to give the reader some indication of the statistical uncertainty of the plotted curve (this has been done, for example, for the survival curves in Chapter 20).

Survival curves can be compared by statistical tests to see whether, for example, the curves are different for one group receiving a certain type of treatment compared with an untreated group, but we shall not discuss such tests in detail here.

If you have any familiarity with spreadsheet programs for personal computers, you will see that it is really quite easy to perform a survival analysis using such a program. Times, events and censorings are entered in separate columns, and three simple repeated formulae calculate the n_i, L_i and S_i for each line.

THE DIFFERENCE BETWEEN RISK AND RATE

Another way to analyse the data in the above example would be to calculate the rate of infection per person-month, just as we did in the example in Chapter 6. Let us first look rather more stringently at the definition of rates.

Rate is really an instantaneous measure, and as such it is rather an abstraction. It could be compared to the actual value on the speedometer of a car. Even if the needle is pointing at 72 km/hour right now, that does not mean that we will travel exactly 72 km during the next hour – it is just the speed at which we are driving at the moment.

Rate is always calculated as the number who fall ill as a proportion of those who are susceptible at that precise moment in time, which means that if people are infected and becoming immune, then the number of susceptible individuals in the denominator is decreasing with time (in epidemiological literature, the number of susceptible subjects is often called the 'number at risk').

For example, let us assume that herpes simplex virus type 1 infects a population of 100 children at a constant rate. Initially they are all susceptible, and during the first year of our study we diagnose 12 cases. This means that the risk of contracting herpes during a period of 1 year is 12/100 = 0.12, or 12%, which might seem reasonable. However, if we extrapolate to 10 years it appears that the risk of contracting herpes will be 120%, which cannot be true, since a risk can never be higher than 100%.

As has been mentioned previously, a figure for a risk must always include the time period we are considering. If exposure to a pathogen is continuous, then the probability of observing an infection in a study subject will obviously be greater the longer he or she is followed. In an influenza epidemic lasting from November until February, the risk of becoming infected in November will be lower than the risk of becoming infected at any time during the 4-month epidemic.

If we instead calculate the rate, this problem of having to state the time period of observation can be avoided. Assume that the 12 cases in the above herpes example appear evenly over the year. We shall then follow 100 children for 1 month, but after this one child will have had an infection with herpes type 1. We then follow 99 susceptible individuals for another month, but after that one more will have had the disease. We thus follow 98 children for the third month, and so on.

The total number of person-months added during the 1-year study will thus be 100 + 99 + 98 + 97 + . . . + 90 + 89 = 1134. This means that the rate is 12/1134 = 0.0106, or 1.06% per person-month. Just as in the example with speed, it does not matter which time unit we choose to measure rate – a speed of 72 km/hour is the same as 1.2 km/minute, or 20 m/second. A rate of 1.06% per person-month is thus equal to $12 \times 1.06 = 12.7\%$ per person-year. We can see that the rate per year is slightly higher than the risk of contracting herpes during a period of 1 year. (Mathematically, this is due to the fact that the denominator for calculation of risk is the original 100 children, whereas the denominator in the rate calculation decreases with the number of children who contract herpes infection during the year.)

The way to get from rate to risk is by using the following formula:

$$\text{Risk} = 1 - \exp^{-\text{Rate} \times \text{time}}$$

where time is measured in the same units for risk and for rate. The risk of contracting a herpes type 1 infection during a period of 10 years in this example would thus be as follows:

$$\text{Risk over 10 years} = 1 - \exp^{-0.127 \times 10} = 1 - 0.28 = 0.72 = 72\%$$

or slightly less than 100%, which appears reasonable, as a few people will always escape infection. (Parenthetically, we can also see that the risk during a period of 1 year is as follows:

$$1 - \exp^{-0.127 \times 1} = 1 - 0.88 = 0.12 \text{ or } 12\%$$

just as we calculated at the outset.)

Many diseases are so rare that the difference between risk and rate becomes negligible. If one out of every 100 000 individuals in a country contracts meningococcal meningitis each year, this does not appreciably change the number at risk, and in this case the risk *and* the rate are both 1/100 000 per year.

To return to the hepatitis A example that we have spent the greater part of this chapter analysing by survival methods. The number of person-months in this study is easily calculated from the second table in the example – the total for all 12 subjects is 58. There were three people infected with hepatitis A virus, and the rate thus becomes 3/58 cases per person-month = 0.05, meaning that there was slightly less than a 5% risk of becoming infected during each month in the high-endemic country. If we multiply this figure by 12 we get 0.62, which is the rate of infection per person-year.

This is also an interesting figure, but it fails to reveal the important fact shown in the Kaplan–Meier graph above, namely that there were no infections at all during the first 3 to 4 months. When rates are being calculated as above, it is always assumed that the incidence rate remains constant over time. The survival analysis gives much more information about changes in rate over time.

SUMMARY

The distribution of time periods until some positive or negative event occurs is best studied in cohorts of subjects and analysed by survival analysis. This is especially true if the time periods are long, giving considerable problems with losses to follow-up during the study. In survival analysis, the time in the cohort is divided into smaller units, such as months or years, and for each time unit the number of subjects who could experience the event under study (e.g. the number of subjects still in the cohort who are susceptible) is compared with the actual number of events during the time period (e.g. the number of cases). This ratio becomes an estimate of the incidence during this time unit. All of the time units are then put together to obtain an overall survival curve, which is often plotted as a Kaplan–Meier graph.

Figures for risks always, either implicitly or explicitly, refer to a certain time period. By calculating rates, it becomes possible to obtain an incidence measure that is independent of time period. However, when rates are calculated as the number of events per person-month or person-year, a constant incidence rate is assumed, and variations in incidence over time become more evident from a Kaplan–Meier plot.

Chapter 11
Mathematical models
for epidemics

Here we are introduced to the mathematical background to the theory of epidemics. A simple model for an epidemic is presented, and the restrictions of such models are discussed. The importance of contact patterns and immunity for the shape of an epidemic – or endemic – is underlined.

One of the perpetual dreams of mankind has been to be able to predict the future. The regular recurrence of epidemics, and the similar shapes of consecutive epidemics of a disease have long tempted people of a mathematical inclination to construct some kind of model. One need only look at the graph for reported cases of measles in England and Wales before the introduction of vaccine (see Figure 11.1) to see that there is a very clear pattern here.

With the exception of 1948, the epidemic peaks evidently occur every second year, and the highest number of cases during an epidemic always seems to be in the first quarter of the year. The curves for the two periods 1950–51 and 1952–53 are strikingly similar. Surely there must be some way of describing this pattern in mathematical terms – to make some kind of model of measles incidence, which could then be used to predict future epidemics.

If this way of thinking about infectious diseases in terms of models seems somewhat far-fetched, one only needs to consider all of the results of similar models that we encounter daily in other circumstances.

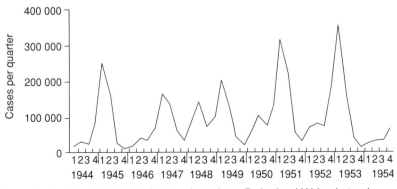

Figure 11.1 Quarterly reported cases of measles in England and Wales during the period 1944–54.

One of the most complex examples is given by the weather forecasts, which are made using supercomputers, where large systems of equations are linked to huge libraries of previous meteorological patterns. The present situation is compared with these data, and the most probable future course is then calculated. Another ramification has been to try to predict sociological developments, for although the future actions of an individual may be impossible to foresee, it might be feasible to say something about how large groups of people will behave. This type of model is best represented by the economic forecasts that are regularly made by banks and financial institutions. The fact that these forecasts rarely turn out to be the same as the actual economic development does not seem to diminish their news value – a good example of our insatiable need to see into the future.

In contrast to the prophecies of cards or crystal balls, predictions about the future that are based on a scientific way of thinking are often phrased in mathematical terms. This can make them difficult to understand for the non-mathematician, and it also lends them an air of exactitude that they seldom merit. No model will be better than the assumptions on which it was built, and these assumptions are usually quite easy to understand and question, even if the formulae look offputting. It is sometimes difficult to see the exact assumptions underlying the model, but in any good publication they should be stated clearly.

Models can be useful for other purposes than predictions. By giving a simplified picture of a development, where less important factors have been removed, they can aid us in understanding complex contexts. Consequently they may also help us to realize which factors are the most important determinants of the development, and therefore which factors we should study more closely and try to measure more precisely.

Finally, models make quite good tools for teaching infectious disease epidemiology.

BASIC REPRODUCTIVE RATE

We have already come across the concept of reproductive rate in Chapter 2, and we have seen that it measures the potential for an infection to spread in a population.

Figure 11.2 shows the schematic spread of an infectious disease.

The disease is brought into the group by the person at the left-hand border. He infects one person, who in turn infects two others. One of these does not spread the infection, but the other infects one more individual, and so on. We can see that the average number of individuals directly infected by each case is $(1 + 2 + 0 + 1 + 3 + 2 + 1 + 1 + 2 + 1 + 2)/10 = 1.5$.

The *basic reproductive rate* is called R_0 (pronounced 'R nought') and has a strict definition:

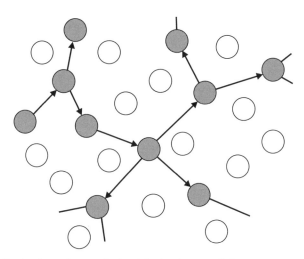

Figure 11.2   A schematic spread of an infection in a population.

R_0 is the average number of individuals directly infected by an infectious case during his or her entire infectious period, when he or she enters a totally susceptible population.

The reason for including the clause 'totally susceptible population' in the definition of basic reproductive rate is as follows. If the disease is one that confers immunity after infection, then the number of susceptible individuals in the population will decrease with time, and more and more of an infectious person's contacts will be with people who are already immune. The actual reproductive rate thus decreases as the infection spreads, but the *basic* rate is unaffected by this.

Obviously R_0 is rather an abstraction. In order to calculate an average R_0, we would first introduce an infectious case into a population and count the number of secondary cases. We would then have to take the original case out of the population again, reset the rest of the population back to its original totally susceptible state, introduce a new first case, count secondary cases, and so on. Thus the strict definition above becomes quite theoretical, but we can usually obtain a good estimate of R_0 by counting the secondary cases so long as the number of already immune contacts is negligible.

Also note the words 'directly infected' in the definition. In Figure 11.2, one could regard the person at the left-hand border as being responsible for all of the subsequent infections. However, it is just the true secondary infections of each case that are counted. In real life, it would of course almost never be known exactly how the disease spread in the group.

Once an epidemic is under way, the current reproductive rate is usually denoted simply by R.

If a new disease enters a population, what is its probability of spreading? From the above reasoning, it may not come as a total surprise that the necessary condition for an epidemic is that R_0 is greater than 1. This means that every infected person on average infects more than one new person. In fact, the three possible situations are as follows:

- $R_0 < 1 \Rightarrow$ the disease will eventually disappear;
- $R_0 = 1 \Rightarrow$ the disease will become endemic;
- $R_0 > 1 \Rightarrow$ there will be an epidemic.

If R_0 is < 1, then every new wave of infection in the population will consist of fewer individuals than the one before, and eventually the disease will die out. If R_0 is equal to 1, then there will be approximately the same number of people infected all the time, which is the definition of an endemic, and if R_0 is > 1, there will be an ever increasing number of infected individuals.

Now let us see what happens if people become immune after infection. Let us assume that R_0 for a disease is 2 (i.e. in the beginning every case infects on average two susceptible individuals). As time goes by, more and more people are becoming immune, and at some time point half of the population will have become immune to the disease. This means that of all the contacts an infectious case will have with other people, only half will actually transmit the infection, and R will have fallen from the original value of 2 to 1. As even more individuals become immune, the actual R will continue to fall below 1, and the epidemic will eventually die out.

This line of reasoning has important implications for the issue of vaccination coverage. If, instead of letting the natural infection gradually increase the proportion of immune individuals as above, we vaccinate the population against a disease, what proportion of the population must be immunized in order to prevent an epidemic? If the basic reproduction rate is R_0, this means that on average R_0 contacts will be infected by someone who has the infection. Suppose we have a disease for which $R_0 = 4$ in a susceptible population. In the unvaccinated natural stage, a primary case of disease will thus infect four people. However, if 25% of the population have already been immunized against the disease, then one of the four people who *should* have become infected by the primary case will escape infection. (Remember that we are always talking about averages when considering R_0, and on average one in every four potential secondary cases will be protected by the immunization.) Thus in this partly immunized population the index case will only infect three people on average.

If half of the population has been immunized, then the primary case will only infect two people, and if 75% of the population have been immunized, there will only be one secondary case, on average. We can see that if 75% have been immunized, there will be a kind of endemic situation in the early stages, with each infectious case infecting one more on average. (After the infection has spread for a while, the actual R will of course drop below 1, since more and more individuals are also becoming naturally immunized.)

Now comes the crucial bit. If *more* than three-quarters of the population have been immunized, then right from the beginning there will be less than one new case per infectious individual on average, and the epidemic cannot even begin to spread.

This example was for an R_0 of 4. We could generalize the argument to any R_0. Assume that the proportion p of the population have already been immunized. Of the R_0 individuals who *should* have become infected by this person bringing the disease into the population, $p \times R_0$ will thus escape infection. Therefore the number of people who will become infected by the primary case is, on average, $R_0 - p \times R_0$. If we want to be certain that the disease will not spread in an epidemic fashion, we want the number of secondary cases from this one infectious primary case to be less than 1, on average. What does this tell us about p, the level of immunization required?

The number of secondary cases $R_0 - p \times R_0$ should be less than 1:

$$R_0 - p \times R_0 < 1$$

which is equal to

$$R_0 - 1 < p \times R_0$$

or:

$$p > (R_0 - 1)/R_0 = 1 - 1/R_0$$

Here we have shown a fundamental formula for vaccination protection. In order to prevent epidemics of a disease, the proportion of the population that must be immunized is higher than 1 minus the inverse of the basic reproductive rate.

Note that I have used the word 'immunized' instead of 'vaccinated' in the above paragraphs. This is because not all vaccines are 100% efficient – all vaccinated people may not have become immunized. Thus the vaccination level may have to be higher than the immunization level.

It is very important to understand that this immunization level will not prevent *all* secondary cases of the disease. Unless coverage is 100%, there will always be some secondary – and even tertiary – cases from newly introduced infectious sources. What we have shown is that with this immunization level, there cannot be any real epidemics in this population. Any little 'micro-epidemic' arising round an infectious case will soon die out on its own.

Consider measles as an example. In a susceptible Western population, R_0 for this disease has been shown to be around 15 (i.e. every case of measles will infect 15 other people on average). Then the formula predicts that if we want to prevent measles epidemics, more than $1 - 1/15 = 0.94$ or 94% of the population must be immunized.

The level of immunity in a population which prevents epidemics (even if some transmissions may still occur) is called *herd immunity*. The higher R_0 is for a disease, the higher the proportion of the population that will have to be vaccinated to achieve herd immunity, which seems rather logical.

These calculations could seem somewhat theoretical, but almost exactly this line of reasoning was used when the World Health Organization devised a strategy to eradicate smallpox in the 1960s, and when there was a resolution to eradicate measles from the USA at about the same time.

WHAT DETERMINES R_0?

I have repeatedly stressed above that R_0 is always an average value, where the number of transmissions from each infectious person is averaged. This means that if there are large differences in the rate of spread within different subgroups of the population, the average R_0 will be quite meaningless. The concept of R_0 finds its greatest use in the description of diseases that are spread broadly among individuals meeting more or less at random.

The basic formula that gives the actual value of R_0 is as follows:

$$R_0 = \beta \times \kappa \times D$$

where β is the risk of transmission per contact (i.e. basically the attack rate), κ is the number of such contacts that an average person in the population would normally have per time unit (in the absence of any disease), and D is the duration of infectivity of an infected person, measured in the same time units as κ was.

We shall now dissect this formula to see what it means. β, the transmission risk per contact, is of course different for different diseases and different types of contacts. Taking HIV infection as an example, we could say that β for the contact 'shaking hands' is zero, as the infection is not transmitted in that way. For sexual intercourse, β is probably somewhere between 0.001 and 0.1, and for the contact 'blood transfusion', which could be seen as a very close contact between the donor and the recipient, β is virtually 1.0.

Table 4.3 from Hope Simpson's studies of childhood diseases gave examples of attack rates for three diseases:

Measles	0.80
Chicken-pox	0.72
Mumps	0.38

In this case 'contact' should be taken to mean 'being siblings in the same household', and it is probable that the β values would be lower for more casual contacts.

Many public health measures to prevent the spread of infections aim at decreasing β – for example, using a condom, wearing a face mask, or washing one's hands.

κ– the average number of contacts a person has per time unit, is of course also different for different transmission routes. In a measles outbreak in a school, it could be the average number of children any child passes each day. The R_0 for a sexually transmitted infection would depend on the number of new partners per month or year. To estimate the spread of a common cold, one would need to know the number of people one would normally pass within sneezing distance – or even just shake hands with – during one day.

Isolation of cases is a public health measure which aims at decreasing κ, even though it often may not be very effective. Public campaigns that recommend people to have fewer sexual partners are another example.

D, the average duration of infectivity, is a biological constant for any disease. With antibiotics, it is often possible to shorten D, and this is one of the instances where infectious disease epidemiology is rather unique, as treatment of ill people actually reduces the risk to others. However, it should be noted that this is not true for all infections. For example, antibiotics for a salmonella infection do not appear to influence the length of time for which a person remains a carrier.

The above formula is really quite trivial – the more infectious a disease is, and the more people a case meets, and the longer he or she is infective, the higher the rate of secondary infections will be. However, it is often enlightening to dissect an epidemic situation in this formal way.

For example, imagine that a sexually transmitted infection in a certain population has an R_0 of 1.2, and would therefore build up to an epidemic. If we could persuade just one-quarter of all couples to use a condom, and assume that β would be 0 in those contacts, R would fall to 0.9 and the infection would eventually disappear.

AN APPROXIMATE FORMULA FOR R_0

From these discussions it should be clear that the higher the R_0 value is for an infection that is spread broadly in society by everyday contacts, the greater the risk will be of encountering this infection early in life. If the transmission risk is high, and if many people are infectious, the chances are that many children will be infected. In fact, it is precisely those infections which have a high R_0 and confer long immunity that we call childhood diseases, since practically everyone is exposed to them and infected in childhood, but subsequently protected from disease.

For such diseases a simple approximate formula exists to estimate R_0 from a knowledge of average age at infection[1]:

$$R_0 = 1 + L/A$$

where L is the average life span of the individuals in the population, and A is the average age at infection. You can see that if the average life expectancy at birth is 70 years, a disease for which the average age at infection is 7 years would have an R_0 of 11. If measles has an R_0 of 15 in Western countries as stated above, then this formula should give an average age at infection of just under 5 years, which seems reasonable.

A SIMPLE MODEL

Most of the mathematical models of infectious diseases that have been published concern childhood diseases (i.e. illnesses that are highly contagious, have short incubation periods and short durations, and confer immunity after infection). We shall look at such a model here, making the following assumptions:

- the population is fixed, (i.e. no one enters and no one leaves or dies);

- the latent period is zero (i.e. people become infectious as soon as they are infected);

- the duration of infectivity is just as long as the clinical disease.

The illness is brought into the group by someone who broke the first rule temporarily, and contracted the illness outside.

We call the size of the population n. At any time, it can be divided into three proportions as follows:

- S, which is the proportion of n that is susceptible;

- I, which is the proportion of n that is currently infected and infectious;

- R, which is the proportion of n that is immune (calling this 'R' is an old custom; it stands for 'resistant'). Do not confuse this 'R' with the one in 'R_0' – they are quite different.

Before the first case is infected, S is obviously equal to 1, since everyone is susceptible, and I and R are both zero. As the epidemic spreads, S will decrease and R will increase. Intuitively, I should first increase and then decrease.

We shall now set up three equations to show how these three proportions will change over time. In doing this, we will use the time derivatives of the proportions. This is written as follows:

$$\frac{dX}{dt}, \text{ where } X \text{ could be } S, I \text{ or } R.$$

If you are unfamiliar with this notation, just read it as 'the rate at which X is currently changing'. If there is a minus sign in front of the derivative, this means that X is currently decreasing. Otherwise it is increasing.

At any time during the epidemic, the three equations will be as follows:

$$\frac{dS}{dt} = -\beta \times \kappa \times S \times I \tag{1}$$

$$\frac{dI}{dt} = \beta \times \kappa \times S \times I - \frac{I}{D} \tag{2}$$

$$\frac{dR}{dt} = \frac{I}{D} \tag{3}$$

Let us look at these equations one at a time. The first one states that the proportion of susceptible individuals is decreasing (minus sign), just as we guessed. However, the actual rate of decrease, $\beta \times \kappa \times S \times I$, deserves an explanation. Look at the $S \times I$ part first. In the population, the following six different types of contacts are possible:

- susceptible meets susceptible;

- susceptible meets infectious;

- susceptible meets resistant (immune);

- infectious meets infectious;

- infectious meets resistant;

- resistant meets resistant.

Obviously, transmission can only occur in the second type (susceptible meets infectious). If all contacts take place completely at random, the proportion of all contacts that occur between members of two groups will be the product of these two groups' respective proportions (i.e. $S \times I$ in this case). To give an example, if 30% of the population belong to the susceptible group, there will be at least one susceptible involved in 30% of all contacts. If a further 10% are infectious, they will represent 10% of all the contacts of the susceptible group, and thus $0.30 \times 0.10 = 0.03$ or 3% of all contacts in the total group will be between susceptible and infectious individuals. (Similarly, $0.30 \times 0.30 = 0.09$ or 9% of all contacts will be between two susceptible individuals, and 1% of all contacts will be between two infectious individuals.)

κ is the average number of contacts any person in the population has, say, per day. Out of all these contacts, just the fraction $S \times I$ will be of the type that could result in a transmission, and $\kappa \times S \times I$ is thus the number of potentially infectious contacts per day. Finally, to obtain the number of transmissions that are actually occurring, we multiply by β, which is the risk of transmission in each of these contacts.

In the second equation, the first term on the right-hand side states that the proportion of infected individuals increases at the same rate as the susceptible individuals are leaving the susceptible pool, which is obvious. However, after time D, an infected person becomes immune, and is taken out of the infectious group, so that if D is equal to 10 days, then 1/10 of all the infected individuals become immune each day. The third equation merely states that the people who leave the infectious group because they become immune are entering the resistant group.

A simpler way to write these formulae is to use difference equations, just as we did in Chapter 10 on survival analysis. They would then appear as follows:

$$S_{t+1} = S_t - \beta \times \kappa \times S_t \times I_t \tag{1}$$

$$I_{t+1} = I_t + \beta \times \kappa \times S_t \times I_t - I_t/D \tag{2}$$

$$R_{t+1} = R_t + I_t/D \tag{3}$$

and this format makes it easy to depict the epidemic using a spreadsheet program.

Assume that the disease has a transmission probability of 0.15 (= β), that individuals in this population have on average 12 contacts per week (= κ), and that the disease lasts for 1 week (= D). As before, the latent period is zero, and the period of infectivity is just as long as the disease span. We start with 1000 people, and introduce one infectious case in week 1. Figure 11.3 shows the number of susceptible individuals remaining in the population each week. (In the calculations for this graph I have let S, I and R denote the proportions as in the above formulae, but then multiplied all numbers by 1000 to convert them into numbers of individuals.)

The epidemic starts off slowly, since there are few infectious cases about. Around week 11, it reaches its maximum incidence rate of some 140 new cases per week, but then it slows down again, this time due to lack of sus-

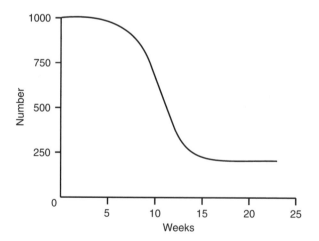

Figure 11.3   Weekly number of susceptible individuals in an imaginary epidemic in a closed population of 1000 people. The epidemic starts with one infectious person being introduced at time zero.

ceptible individuals. By week 16 or 17, the epidemic has subsided. Note that about 200 individuals will escape the infection. The entire course of the epidemic for all three groups is illustrated in Figure 11.4.

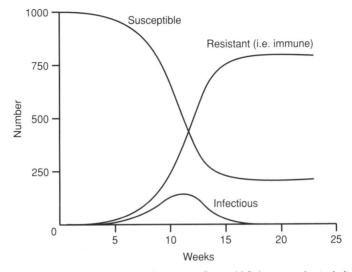

Figure 11.4 The same imaginary epidemic as in Figure 11.3, but now also including weekly numbers of infectious and immune individuals.

The curve for the number of resistant individuals is rather the inverse of the susceptible curve, which makes sense. At the end there will be about 800 people who have become immune. The proportion of the population that is infectious at any one time never exceeds 15%.

Using the basic formula above, $R_0 = \beta \times \kappa \times D$, we would obtain for this epidemic

$$R_0 = 0.15 \times 12 \times 1 = 1.8$$

This shows that even this rather low R_0 can give rise to a substantial epidemic. What happens is that some time around week 11, the actual R falls below 1, and at that point the epidemic starts to tail off.

The fact that not everyone will contract the infection seems counterintuitive. How could 200 of the 1000 people in the above example escape infection when as many as 140 subjects may be infectious at any one time? This lack of total incidence was already noted in smallpox outbreaks in the nineteenth century, and one theory that received much support well into the last century was that the pathogen grew progressively less virulent after repeated passages through individuals. A virus or bacterium would thus be more virulent (i.e. have a higher β value) when passing from the primary case to a secondary one than when passing from generation 10 to generation 11, and this would explain why the outbreak subsided before everyone was affected.

However, the line of reasoning behind the above very simple model makes it clear that this assumption of decreasing virulence is not necessary. Seen from the viewpoint of the epidemic, every infectious subject will be given a certain number of potentially infective exposures to use on other individuals. As the number of immune people increases, more and more of these exposures will be 'thrown away' on non-susceptible individuals, and even if an exposure is used on a susceptible person there is just the probability β that a transmission will actually occur. In some sense, the remaining susceptible individuals will be protected by the large number of immune subjects around them, which is precisely the concept of herd immunity described above.

OBJECTIONS TO THE MODEL

At least two of the basic assumptions underlying this model are seriously unrealistic. The first is that every person in the population will meet every other with equal probability. This may be true for atoms in a mixture of gases, and the formulation of the model above actually derives from chemistry, where the 'law of mass action' describes how substances enter into chemical reactions.

Among people there will always be some contacts that are likely or common, and others that will never occur. One's family is such a 'subgroup' for infectious disease spread, and if you remember the monkey-pox example in Chapter 4, the researchers calculated different attack rates for family contacts and more distant contacts. Other important subgroups are the school, the workplace, one's friends, etc. Differences in age and geographical distances will both have major influences on who meets whom. The fact that the contact pattern in society is far from homogeneous will result in most infections spreading more slowly than the above model predicts. Furthermore, it is quite conceivable that contact patterns change once one becomes ill, as one only has to go to bed for a couple of days with the infection to decrease the number of contacts substantially.

Another problem is that the epidemic itself may well influence the contact pattern. The most difficult thing to model with regard to HIV spread is to what extent the public's changing habits in the face of the epidemic will themselves lead to the epidemic taking another course.

The second unrealistic assumption is that only one type of contact exists, with a given β. As discussed briefly above, diseases may spread along different routes with varying degrees of transmission risk. If subgroups of the population have very different contact modes, there can be very different outcomes of introduction of a disease into these groups. With regard to HIV, anal intercourse and blood-to-blood contact through the sharing of needles carry a higher β than vaginal intercourse. This implies that in a group of homosexual men, or a group of intravenous drug users, there may be a higher risk of epidemic spread than in a non-drug-using heterosexual subgroup of the population, even at the same contact rate.

Again, this takes us back to the sociology of infectious diseases. The potential for an epidemic lies not only with the biological constants of the disease (e.g. transmission risk or duration), but also just as much with the way in which society is organized (e.g. how we travel, the size of our families, the division of the school year, the density of the population, etc.). Many of the epidemics that in the past were perceived as 'new' diseases probably owed their emergence to changing contact patterns (e.g. faster intercontinental travel, increasing population density, etc.). Since the human race has been mixing with its bacteria and viruses for at least a couple of hundred thousand years, the probability of new pathogens suddenly emerging should be rather low. However, it seems to be a historical fact that we fail to see how we change, and how that change gives ground for disease spread.

This is with all probability also true for the future. Right now there are pathogens out there leading their quiet lives, waiting for us humans to change our ways of life so that they will find an ecological niche in our society.

THE ROLE OF CHANCE

The way of thinking about infectious diseases described above is *deterministic*. This means that the development and size of an epidemic are always determined by β, κ and D. Every time our model disease in the above graphs is introduced into a susceptible population, the ensuing epidemic will run the same course.

For established epidemics in large populations, a deterministic model may not be too out of place, but it is intuitively clear that chance may play a major role, especially early in an epidemic. If someone with measles came to an island where only a few people were immune, he would start an epidemic according to the deterministic model. However, if he only happened to meet immune individuals before he recovered, there would be no epidemic at all.

Models that take chance into account are described as *probabilistic,* and often become more mathematically complex than deterministic models. They are usually evaluated using a computer, where a simulated epidemic is run many times. Each run creates a different result due to chance, and these results can be averaged to find the most likely course.

For both deterministic and probabilistic modellers, their main problem is the lack of good quantitative data for infectious diseases. With some exceptions, infectious disease epidemiology has made rather few attempts to assess reliable numerical values for transmission rates, and figures for contact rates are even scarcer. Predictions in particular will be very sensitive to exact numbers, and as a general rule one could say that it is much easier to write down the formulae of a model than to collect good data to put into it.

SUMMARY

Models of diseases that spread from person to person rely on the concept of reproduction rate, which is the average number of people infected by one case. This depends on the attack rate of the disease, the frequency of contacts, and the duration of infectivity. If the proportion of immune individuals in a group is high, few contacts will result in transmission, and epidemics will become impossible. This is called herd immunity.

A simple model for a childhood disease consists of three differential equations, and this exhibits a few of the details that are characteristic of such a disease.

The major problem with all infectious disease models is that the contact pattern in the population is often unknown and very complicated to model. This makes it extremely difficult to predict the future course of evolving epidemics.

In the following chapters we shall look at some examples where these specific concepts of infectious disease epidemiology have been studied.

REFERENCES

1. Dietz K. Transmission and control of arbovirus diseases. In: Ludwig D, Cooke KI (eds) *Epidemiology*. Philadelphia, PA: Society for Industrial and Applied Mathematics, 1975: 104–21.

Chapter 12
Detection and
analysis of outbreaks

Here the epidemiology of outbreak investigations is discussed. The importance of case definitions is stressed, and the various types of epidemic curves are presented. Three examples of different outbreak investigations are analysed in some detail.

Almost every investigation of an outbreak of a known or new disease starts with someone noticing an excess of cases. If you look back at Chapter 2, that is almost exactly the definition of an epidemic given by Benenson: 'The occurrence of cases of an illness clearly in excess of expectancy'. The key word here is 'expectancy'. When does one get the feeling that this is more than it should have been? In the previous chapters we have looked at the concepts of risks and rates from different angles, always stressing that such measures need not only a figure for the cases, but also some comparison or denominator. When someone suddenly notices an excess of cases, such formal comparisons are seldom made. Instead, one uses one's general, everyday knowledge and experience, which yield some rather imprecise feeling for what is usual and common and what is not.

Such notions are necessary for any more rigorous investigation to get started. However, one should be very careful not to put too much faith in them, and many misconceptions in medicine – as in human affairs in general – come from uncritical reliance on numbers, without consideration of denominators or control groups. The ominous expression 'no smoke without fire' is a good example.

This concept of a perceived deviation from normal can be carried over into the investigation of outbreaks. In such a situation, it is usually clear that something has happened outside 'expectancy'. The immediate task is to find and describe the cases, and to analyse them for any unexpected pattern. The controlling is supplied by common sense. For example, if we find that 80% of the cases in an outbreak are women, this must be an important piece of information even without further formal analysis, since we know that the expected proportion of women should be around 50%. If we find that all of the cases live in one section of a city, this is an unexpected finding, and would implicate some geographical risk of exposure. As an example of the opposite situation, namely lack of outbreaks, Jenner noted in the late 1700s that milkmaids seldom fell ill with smallpox, and from this observation he proceeded to introduce vaccinia inoculation as a vaccine for smallpox.

METHODS

An analysis of an outbreak always starts with descriptive epidemiology. The three important words here are *time*, *place* and *person*, and the following two questions need to be answered as early as possible in an outbreak.

1. What pathogen is causing the disease?

2. Where is the source?

However, even before these two questions are satisfactorily answered it may sometimes be possible to instigate broad preventive measures for the protection of susceptible individuals, such as recommending the boiling of drinking water, or closing a school.

The first thing one has to do is to decide who is a case and who is not. To this end, one needs a *case definition*, which should include the typical symptoms of the patients in the outbreak. In addition, the time interval over which the illness should have broken out must be specified, because we do not want to include people with similar symptoms from other causes. A typical case definition might be as follows: 'All children in form 3 of the local school who took part in the field trip on 20 November, and who fell ill with vomiting and/or diarrhoea between the evening of the 20th and the evening of the 21st.' The symptoms of the case definition are best assessed from interviews with a couple of cases regarded as typical of the outbreak. These people should also be the first ones to yield samples for microbiological analysis.

As you can see, such a relatively detailed case definition already requires a fairly good overview of the outbreak (group afflicted, times of onset), and often one does not have such a firm picture of the outbreak during the initial phases. It is best to start with a broad tentative case definition, which can be narrowed down as more and more becomes known about the outbreak.

During the following hours or days one attempts to find all the cases of the outbreak, or at least a representative sample. Their sexes and ages should be recorded, as well as information on times of onset, symptoms, times of suspected exposures, and geographical information. If the disease is gastroenteritis, one will try to obtain as detailed a food history as possible. If it is an airborne infection, one will need exact information on the patient's movements during the presumed incubation period.

It is almost always a good idea to develop a questionnaire before the interviews start. In this way, one will remember to ask all the pertinent questions, and if several different investigators are working simultaneously, a questionnaire will ensure that they collect the same information with as little interviewer bias as possible.

The responses from the cases are used to construct graphs of the types discussed in Chapter 3.

Epidemic curve

The date at which each case fell ill is plotted along a horizontal axis in the following manner, where each square denotes a patient as shown in Figure 12.1. (One usually works from a list of cases, where each case has a number. It is often useful to write these numbers in the corresponding squares on the curve, since that will make it easy to move back and forth between the graph and the list.)

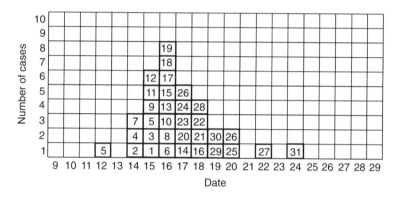

Figure 12.1   An example of a point-source outbreak.

In this particular epidemic, the earliest case occurred on the 12th day of the month, with the incidence being highest on the 16th, and no cases after the 24th. This type of epidemic curve, which is clustered around a peak value, points to a common event when all 31 cases were infected at the same time, and this is a typical example of a *point source outbreak*. You will notice that the first case to be diagnosed was not the first case in time. This is quite common in outbreak investigations, when extended case-finding reveals cases that were not noticed or not reported initially (or in other words, the index case was not the primary case).

Case 5 should correspond to the shortest possible incubation time for the disease, and case 31 to the longest one. If we already have a suspect infectious event, we could guess which disease this is from our knowledge of the incubation time of different diseases.

Another type of epidemic curve is shown in Figure 12.2 below.

Such a pattern is more indicative of a *continuous source*, where for example drinking water is being polluted, or some foodstuff is being continuously contaminated.

In a situation involving person-to-person spread, the epidemic curve will appear as shown in Figure 12.3.

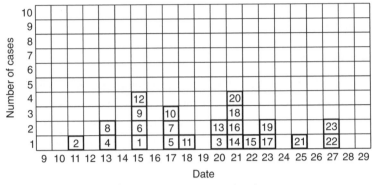

Figure 12.2 An example of a continuous-source outbreak.

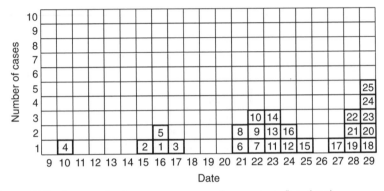

Figure 12.3 An example of a person-to-person (or propagated) outbreak.

Here the person who fell ill on the 10th day of the month probably infected the group of people who fell ill between the 15th and 17th, and this group again caused a new group of cases around the 23rd. The interval between successive waves of disease seems to be about 7 days, but you can see that the variation around this average value will make the cyclic epidemic pattern disappear after a couple of waves. As was pointed out in Chapter 2, this interval is called the serial interval, and it is often shorter than the incubation period. This is evident if one considers that the primary case could well have been infectious several days before he became ill on the 10th day of the month, which means that the secondary cases had an incubation period of more than the 5 to 8 days indicated by the above curve.

Geography

In many outbreaks, it may be enlightening to plot all of the cases on a map to see whether there is evidence of clustering. However, in modern society few people spend all day in the same place, and it often becomes quite difficult to decide which place should be plotted (e.g home, workplace, holiday resort). This is a major problem for the use of Geographical Information Systems (GIS) analysis in epidemiology, a new tool that is becoming increasingly popular.

GIS methods might be very useful for studying rabies in racoons or factors that influence tick-borne encephalitis virus prevalence in ticks, since neither animal moves around very much, but humans can travel quickly over large distances. Most routine surveillance systems only record where the patient was diagnosed, which may be a long distance from where they were actually infected. Early maps of the international spread of AIDS were more like depictions of the major airline routes than of any epidemiological pattern.

A good counter-example concerns water-borne outbreaks in a community. In such outbreaks it can often be very informative to plot a map of the water distribution network over the map of cases – just as Snow did 150 years ago.

Age and sex

A third plot that may yield information on aetiology is a population pyramid of the cases. Figure 12.4 is a rather extreme example which builds on a real outbreak that occurred in Sweden several years ago.

This graph shows the different age groups on the vertical axes, and the number of cases in each group as squares to the left and right. The disease was gastroenteritis, and there was a rather prolonged epidemic. What could cause this peculiar pattern, with cases among children, young adult women and old people? The answer was canned baby food infected with salmonella. The babies obviously contracted the infection from eating baby food, their mothers from tasting it before feeding them, and the old age pensioners from buying baby food for dental or economic reasons.

All of these curves only show the patterns among cases, without any controls or denominators. However, as soon as we believe that we can see a pattern among the cases, we can go on to a more rigorous analysis, by contracting those people who seem to have been exposed at the outbreak, but who did not become ill. By asking those controls carefully about their exposure, it becomes possible to implicate a specific source much more reliably, just as we did in Chapters 4 and 5.

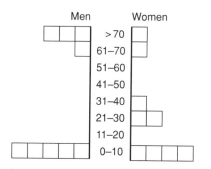

Figure 12.4 Simplified curve showing age and sex distribution of an outbreak of gastroenteritis in Sweden.

THREE REAL-LIFE EXAMPLES

A hepatitis B outbreak

A good example of an outbreak investigation comes from a small epidemic of hepatitis B among diabetes patients in the USA[1].

As always, the investigation was sparked by someone noticing an increased number of cases. During a 10-month period in 1989–90, 20 cases of acute hepatitis B were diagnosed among the patients in a hospital, compared with four during the previous year. This seems like a sixfold increase in incidence calculated on a yearly basis, provided that the denominator remained constant (i.e. there were constant rates of admission and discharge during the two periods).

The 20 patients during the 10-month period were initially defined as the cases, and their medical records were consulted for possible connections. It was found that 18 of these patients had diabetes, that all but one of them were male, and that they had all been admitted to a single medical ward at some time during the 6 months preceding their illness. Common sense alone allows one to decide that it is improbable that these three findings should have arisen by chance.

The next step was to look actively for more cases. All of the more than 500 patients who had been admitted to the ward at any time during 1989 and who were still alive at the time of the study were approached and requested to provide a blood sample. Seven more cases were detected in this way. An interesting point mentioned in the paper is that only seven of the 27 cases (26%) had had any symptoms of an acute hepatitis B infection. There must have been a continuing strategy of testing for hepatitis markers in this hospital, or it is unlikely that the outbreak would have been discovered.

The resulting epidemic curve for the entire 14-month outbreak is shown in Figure 12.5.

The incubation period for hepatitis B is 2 to 6 months, and the serial interval is perhaps 1 month shorter. The epidemic curve could thus describe a person-to-person spread, with the primary case being diagnosed in March 1989,

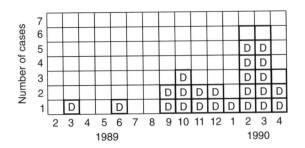

Figure 12.5 Epidemic curve for a prolonged outbreak of hepatitis B on a ward. D represents diabetes patients. (*Source*: Polish et al.[1].)

the secondary case diagnosed in June 1989, and 25 tertiary and higher-order cases thereafter.

The risk factors for becoming infected (other than having diabetes) were explored in a retrospective cohort study, including all patients with diabetes who had been admitted to the ward after the primary case described above had been discharged. In total, 23 patients were the cases shown in Figure 12.5, and 37 patients were still susceptible to hepatitis B infection. The relative risk of becoming infected was calculated for a number of factors, such as age, sex, race, date of hospitalization, location of beds in the ward, other behavioural risks, etc. The only factor that showed a strong association with infection was the use of a spring-loaded device for taking capillary blood samples, for which the 2×2 table was as follows:

	Infected	Susceptible	
Spring device used	23	32	55
Spring device not used	0	5	5
	23	37	60

The risk of infection in the patients who had samples taken with the spring-loaded device was thus $23/55 = 0.42$, compared with $0/5 = 0$ in the group who had not had their capillary samples taken in this way. The probability that this difference would occur by chance is 0.08 according to Fisher's exact test.

The investigators then proceeded to perform a case–control study comparing the three non-diabetic patients who contracted hepatitis with a random sample of 20 non-diabetic, still susceptible patients from the population of all patients who had been hospitalized during the year. When analysing for the exposure 'capillary test taken by spring-loaded device', they obtained the following result:

	Infected	Susceptible	
Spring device used	3	0	3
Spring device not used	0	20	20
	3	20	60

The OR cannot be calculated, due to the zeros, but Fisher's exact test gives a probability of 0.006 that all of the three infected patients should have been exposed to this risk, compared with none of the 20 others, just by chance.

The authors conclude that minute amounts of infected blood could have remained on the device, which was used on consecutive patients, and that this was the probable source of infection. The first case above was a hepatitis B carrier, and the second was a long-term patient on the ward, who was tested for capillary blood glucose regularly, and who could have acted as a 'reservoir' for the spread to other patients.

Lyme disease and ticks

A more protracted example of an outbreak investigation, and one which concerned a new disease, comes from the analysis of early data on Lyme disease.[2] This investigation started in 1975, when several mothers observed that a high number of children in a small, rural area of Connecticut were diagnosed as having juvenile rheumatoid arthritis, which is a rare disease. This observation was followed by a retrospective analysis of 51 cases in the area in early 1976. On four country roads, one child in 10 had the disease, and in that area there were six families who had had more than one case.

Quite early in the investigations, suspicion was directed towards arthropod bites as the aetiology of the disease, and especially tick bites. (If you think that ticks are insects, you are mistaken: they are arachnids.) A prospective study was initiated to run through 1977, which attempted to collect all cases of this new 'Lyme disease' diagnosed in an area of 12 communities on both sides of the Connecticut River.

All physicians and visiting nurses in the area were asked to report cases to the investigators at Yale University, and if possible to refer the patients to them. No laboratory test for the disease was available at the time, so the case definition was entirely clinical, based on the appearance of a typical exanthema, or on brief but recurrent aseptic arthritis.

A total of 43 patients were reported during the year. There was of course no way to ascertain the completeness of the reporting, but 41 of the 55 participating physicians reported at least one case. A chart plotting the epidemic is shown in Figure 12.6.

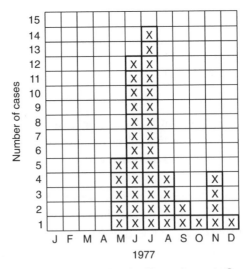

Figure 12.6 Epidemic curve for an outbreak of Lyme disease in Connecticut in 1977. (*Source:* Steere et al.[2].)

It can be seen that the cases start appearing in May, the incidence peaks in early summer, and there are still cases diagnosed during the autumn. The months of June and July account for 60% of the cases.

The most striking finding emerged when the patients were divided into those living east and west of the Connecticut River. There were 35 cases on the east side, and only eight on the west side. In order to assess the value of this information, we need denominators. If there were many more people living on the east side, this could explain the difference in numbers. However, there were 12 400 residents in the communities on the east side, and 60 300 residents on the west side. The risks of disease during the year were thus 2.8 and 0. 13 per 1000 residents, respectively. The relative risk can be calculated to be 21, and an approximate 95% confidence interval is obtained from the formula in Chapter 5. The error factor would be as follows:

$$EF = \exp^{1.96\sqrt{1/a + 1/b}}$$

where $a = 35$ and $b = 8$ (both figures should really be greater than 10 for the formula to be quite valid, but we are just obtaining a rough estimate here),

$$EF = \exp^{1.96\sqrt{1/8 + 1/35}} = 2.2$$

and the lower limit is thus $21/2.2 = 9.5$, which is well above unity. The male : female sex ratio of the cases was $1.2 : 1$, so this did not yield much additional information. Half of the cases were in children aged 15 years or younger, and only one patient was over 50 years old.

All of the findings presented so far fit in rather nicely with the hypothesis of an arthropod vector (especially a non-flying one). The incidence curve correlates well with the life cycle of arthropods, the geographical division by the river could be explained by differing densities of the vector, and the excess of cases in children could be due to the fact that they spend more time out of doors. However, there are many possible biases to be considered.

1. Seasonal variations in incidence are seen for many diseases, and factors such as dietary habits or amounts of allergens in the environment could well vary in such a way as to cause patterns similar to the one in the above curve.

2. The geographical difference could be due to increased clinical awareness among the doctors on the east side of the river.

3. There could be genetic differences between the populations on either side of the river.

4. The age pattern could be due to worried parents consulting physicians about symptoms in their children, but disregarding similar symptoms in themselves.

Next, the investigators performed a case–control study. For each of the 32 patients who were diagnosed between June and September, two neighbourhood controls were chosen, matched with regard to sex and child/adult. (It is not clear from the article why controls were not selected for all of the cases.) The cases and controls were interviewed about a list of possible risk factors, such as the size of their plot, types of outside activities, pets and farm animals, and recollection of arthropod bites in 1977.

Significantly more cases than controls reported tick bites. The former also reported having seen ticks on their pet animals more often than the latter. Even this finding could be due to confounding. If the real risk factor was something else that one would encounter in the wild, then the group of people who reported a tick bite would probably contain a higher proportion of people who spent a large amount of time out of doors, and who would thus be at higher risk of being exposed to the real risk factor. The tick bite would then be a marker of risk behaviour, and not the real cause.

However, at the same time as this investigation was performed, another group measured the density of the tick *Ixodes scapularis* east and west of the river, and found it to be about 15 times more prevalent on wild animals on the east side[3]. All of this pointed to an aetiological role for bites from this tick, and a few years later the spirochaete *Borrelia burgdorferi* was isolated from these ticks and found to be related to a number of clinical symptoms in humans.

Legionnaires' disease

On 21–24 July 1976, the American Legion, Department of Pennsylvania (a congregation of war veterans), held a convention in a hotel in Philadelphia. On 2 August it became clear that there was an outbreak of severe pneumonia of unknown aetiology among the participants, and the Pennsylvania Department of Health started an investigation[4]. A case was defined as someone who had either attended the convention, or entered the hotel after 1 July, *and* who had onset of the following symptoms between 1 July and 18 August:

- cough and fever $\geq 38.90°C$; or

- any fever and X-ray verified pneumonia.

One can see that the clinical case definition is rather wide, and that it will probably include pneumonias of other aetiologies. Moreover, the time period in the epidemiological case definition starts well before the known outbreak, to ensure that early cases were not missed. This would be particularly important if the disease was spread from person to person and had an incubation period of the order of weeks.

Cases were actively sought across the entire state of Pennsylvania, with public health nurses searching hospitals for hospitalized participants, and the public being invited to report cases on a telephone hotline. In total, 182 patients who fulfilled the criteria of the case definition were found, of whom 29 individuals died from the disease, giving a case fatality rate of 16%. A total of 149 of these patients had attended the convention, and another nine had attended other conventions in the hotel just before or just after the Legionnaires' meeting; 84 patients had stayed in the hotel for at least one night. Figure 12.7 illustrates the epidemic curve.

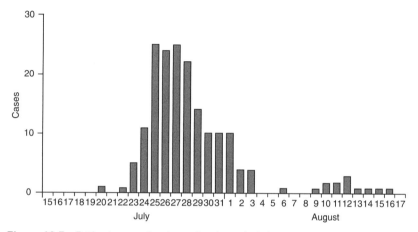

Figure 12.7 Epidemic curve for the outbreak in which Legionnaires' disease was first described. (*Source*: Fraser et al.[4].)

Disregarding the trickle of cases in August, this epidemic curve looks like almost a textbook example of a point source outbreak.

There was no evidence of similar outbreaks linked to other hotels in the area during this time, or of any general increase in pneumonia mortality in Pennsylvania, but the state-wide search for more cases identified 39 additional patients who met the clinical criteria, but who had not been in the hotel. However, they had been within one block of the hotel during the time period of the case definition.

In total, 142 cases (78%) were men, which is not surprising since this was a veterans' meeting. For the same reason, the age distribution was rather skewed towards higher ages.

This is the straightforward time–place–person description of the outbreak. The significance of the right-skewed age distribution cannot be assessed since we do not know the age distribution of all of the people who came to the convention. The investigators tried to distribute a questionnaire to all participants, and received a reply from 84% of them. From these forms they could calculate age-specific attack rates (bringing in a denominator!). These are shown in Table 12.1.

The attack rate evidently increased with age. It was also higher for delegates than for other people attending the convention.

Table 12.1 Attack rate by age during an outbreak of Legionnaire's disease. (*Source*: Fraser *et al.*[4])

Age group (years)	Cases	Total	Attack rate (%)
< 40	6	160	3.8
40–49	20	392	5.1
50–59	52	843	6.2
60–69	31	315	9.8
≥ 70	16	130	12.3
Total	125	1849	6.8

If 'visiting the hotel' was taken to be the time of exposure, the incubation time for all but two cases could be estimated to be between 2 and 10 days.

On 17 August a telephone interview was undertaken with 113 cases and 147 controls. The subjects were asked about their movements during the four days, and since cases had occurred among people who did not even enter the hotel, the subjects were asked to specify how much time they had spent in the lobby or on the pavement outside the hotel.

In total, 50% of the cases had stayed in the convention hotel, compared only 35% of the controls. This difference was significant. Furthermore, the cases had spent almost twice as much time in the lobby, on average, as had the controls. Among the individuals who watched the Legion parade on 23 July, cases were more likely than controls to have stood on the pavement directly in front of the hotel.

The possibility of person-to-person spread was also examined in a case–control study in which: 59 room-mates of 52 cases were compared with 69 room-mates of 68 controls. Five room-mates from each group (8.5 and 7.2%, respectively) had themselves become ill. This difference is small and statistically non-significant, and it shows that person-to-person spread was unlikely. In addition, no relatives of cases were infected after the latter had returned home.

All of this evidence pointed to an airborne agent for this infection, which must have been most abundant in the lobby and directly outside the hotel. In fact, simultaneously with this investigation, the bacterium *Legionella* was being isolated in the laboratory, and a serological test for infection was also used in the epidemiological work.

CASE–CASE STUDIES

In the next chapter we shall look at surveillance systems which continually collect data on cases of disease. In some outbreak situations such information could be used for a somewhat different study design, called a *case–case study*.

The best example of such a situation would be outbreaks of salmonella infection. In most industrialized countries, salmonella strains are subtyped in the reference laboratory, either by serotyping or by phage typing. Pulse-field gel electrophoresis is becoming increasingly common, but the old methods are still used for naming the more than 2000 serotypes of salmonella that are known (*S. agona, S. malmoe, S. typhimurium, S. wirchow*, etc.). This sub-typing makes it possible to discover outbreaks against an almost constant background of collective salmonella infections.

In many such outbreaks, data on different exposures are collected for the cases (and sometimes for controls, but that will not concern us here). This continuing collection of exposure data forms the basis for the idea of case–case studies[5]. In the analysis of an on-going outbreak of a certain sal-monella strain, we could use exposure data from a recent outbreak of another strain as a control, instead of having to interview a number of ran-domly selected controls in the present outbreak. Since the source of the new outbreak will almost never be the same as in the previous one, the reports from the cases in the old outbreak should give a good estimate of exposure distribution in the background population (consumption and handling of various food items in this case) for all items except the culprit in that out-break.

The obvious advantage of this approach is that it saves time and effort, since we do not have to search for new controls. The data is already regis-tered and stored in a database at the surveillance centre. It does introduce a bias in that all of the 'controls' were previous salmonella cases, but it also takes care of another bias which is not so easily realized. Our background population for a sample of diagnosed salmonella cases is not really the pop-ulation at large, but rather the subpopulation of people who would visit a doctor when they have gastroenteritis. When population controls are chosen in a regular case–control study, we have no way of ascertaining whether the controls belong to this 'visit-prone' subpopulation. Using the notified cases from a previous outbreak as controls, we know that we are dealing with the right subpopulation in this respect.

The bias whereby all of the cases from the previous outbreak may differ from the general population in some important aspect could be circumvented by mixing cases from several past outbreaks in the pool of controls.

This example concerned gastroenteritis caused by salmonella, but the idea is applicable to outbreaks of other infectious diseases for which subtyping of the pathogen is routinely performed.

SECONDARY CASES

For diseases that are not only due to environmental exposures (food, water, animal contact) but that also spread from person to person, the analysis of an outbreak often becomes complicated. This is especially true if the serial inter-val is very short, so that secondary cases start to appear while there are still primary cases becoming ill. If such secondary cases are misclassified as primary and are also interviewed about exposures, any association between exposure and disease may be diluted and lost. This dilution will be severe, for example, in a food-borne outbreak from a shared meal, since the secondary cases will largely come from the group who did *not* eat the infectious food item in the first round.

One example comes from an outbreak of gastroenteritis caused by Norwalk-like viruses (NLV) in a group of day-care homes in north Stockholm, which was investigated by our unit[6]. Food for all of the day-care homes was supplied by one catering firm. On 2 March 1999, an outbreak of severe vomiting and diarrhoea occurred among the 775 children and staff. The epidemic curve is shown in Figure 12.8. The investigation pointed to the lunch served on 1 March as the likely source, and a cohort study was performed to try to identify the food item responsible. NLV infection has an incubation period of 10–50 hours, so as early as the afternoon of 2 March there may be secondary cases among the patients.

Figure 12.8 is thus a superimposition of two epidemic curves – one of primary cases starting on 1 March, and continuing until 3 or 4 March, and one of secondary cases starting on 2 March (or it may even be three curves – one of primary, one of secondary, and one of tertiary cases). It is impossible to tell for a single case whether it is primary or secondary, so a time line has to be drawn somewhere in the figure. Drawing this vertical line far to the left will ensure that few secondary cases are regarded as primary, but on the other hand will reduce the statistical power of the study. In this study, a primary case was defined as a person who became ill during the first 3 days of the outbreak, and a secondary case as one who became ill between day 4 and day 12. Although there is bound to be some misclassification here, this time was

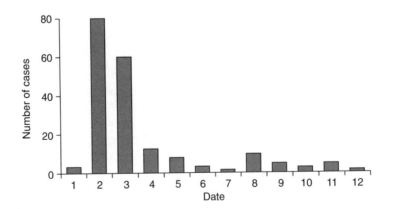

Figure 12.8 Epidemic curve for an outbreak of gastroenteritis caused by Norwalk-like virus in a group of day-care homes in March 1999. Primary and higher-order cases are mixed. (Graph courtesy of Hannelore Götz.)

chosen after an analysis that showed very clear differences in risk factors for disease between these two groups.

SUMMARY

The three most important factors to be characterized in an outbreak analysis are time, place and person. In order to identify the cases for this analysis, one needs a case definition, and this is used to search actively for more cases than the ones who presented themselves. The epidemic curve can give an indication of type of exposure (e.g. point source, extended source, or person to person). In a point source outbreak it is often possible to estimate the common time of exposure, if the disease and its incubation time are known, or conversely to diagnose the disease if the time of exposure is known.

Plots should be constructed not only for the time course of the outbreak, but also for sex and age distribution, and often for the geographical location of the cases.

After the cases have been identified, the probable cause of the outbreak can be investigated by more analytical methods, most often starting with a case–control study. In many instances, the cause will be clear from the outset, since an unexpected increase in the rate of diagnosis of a certain pathogen in the microbiological laboratory will often be what triggered the investigation. However, if the pathogen was previously unknown, epidemiology and microbiology will often need to work hand in hand to reveal the cause.

REFERENCES

1. Polish LB, Shapiro CN, Bauer F et al. Nosocomial transmission of hepatitis B virus associated with the use of a spring-loaded finger-stick device. N Engl J Med 1992; **326**: 721–5.
2. Steere AC, Broderick TF, Malawista SE. Erythema chronicum migrans and Lyme arthritis: epidemiologic evidence for a tick vector. Am J Epidemiol 1978; **108**: 312–21.
3. Wallis RC, Brown SE, Kloter KO, Main AL. Erythema chronicum migrans and Lyme arthritis: field study of ticks. Am J Epidemiol 1978; **108**: 322–7.
4. Fraser DW, Tsai TR, Orenstein W et al. Legionnaires' disease. Description of an epidemic of pneumonia. N Engl J Med 1977; **297**: 1189–97.
5. McCarthy N, Giesecke J. Case–case comparisons to study causation of common infectious diseases. Int J Epidemiol 1999; **28**: 764–8.
6. Götz H, de Jong B, Lindbäck J, Parment PA, Hedlund KO, Torvén M, Ekdahl K. A food-borne gastroenteritis outbreak caused by Norwalk-like virus in 30 day-care centres; epidemiological and microbiological aspects. Scand J Infect Dis 2001, in press.

Chapter 13
Routine surveillance
of infectious diseases

This chapter discusses how data for surveillance are collected and interpreted. Several sources of potential bias are identified.

The previous chapter described the analysis of outbreaks of known or new diseases. In each example the discovery of the outbreak relied on clinical observations, where an unusual aggregation of cases was first noted by physicians or the public. This is a somewhat haphazard mode of detection, and at least for known diseases with an epidemic potential one would feel more secure with an established system that could recognize outbreaks when they occurred.

Since the end of the nineteenth century, many Western countries have thus had systems for the reporting ('notification') of certain infectious diseases. There is also mandatory reporting to the World Health Organization of cases of cholera, yellow fever or plague in any of its member countries. The aim of such reporting systems has always been to discover epidemic outbreaks of infectious disease quickly, and the rationale is that while any one doctor might only see one or two cases of an epidemic, collective reporting at a regional or national level will make it possible to see the full picture.

These notification systems were not instituted as a purely epidemiological exercise, but rather to make possible the rapid application of preventive measures. Exactitude is therefore often less important than speed, and there is seldom time for elaborate epidemiological analysis of data before an action is decided on.

This continuous collection, collation and analysis of data, with or without subsequent action, is often called *surveillance*. A large proportion of studies on infectious disease epidemiology emanates from such surveillance data.

The general principle is that each country has a list of notifiable diseases, which may vary in length from around 10 diseases to over 50 in European countries. Each time a physician diagnoses a patient with one of these diseases, they should report this to a regional or national body. This notification usually goes by mail, but electronic networks are increasingly being used. The amount of information on the notification form varies greatly between countries, but most often includes the diagnosis, date of onset, age, sex, and place of residence of the patient. It may also contain data on symptoms, type of exposure, other similar cases in the vicinity, treatment given and precautions taken.

Another way of collecting incidence data is by reports from the microbiological laboratories. Since for many of the notifiable diseases diagnosis is confirmed by microbiological analysis, standardized reporting from these laboratories will include most such cases. With increasing numbers of laboratories computerizing the handling of samples and reports, such notification also increasingly occurs by direct electronic transmission.

A third data source is discharge notes from hospitals, which should include diagnoses and some data about the patients. The main problems with this source are that it will only contain the most severe cases of the disease (those who were hospitalized), and that the time interval between admission and reporting is often long in a routine system.

For rapid assessment of incidence, more and more countries are also introducing *sentinel* systems ('sentinel' meaning 'guard' or 'watchman'), in which a sample of all general practitioners in the country are asked to report clinical diagnoses of certain diseases at a regional or national level on a weekly basis. The systems usually only include the immediate clinical diagnosis, such as gastroenteritis or influenza-like syndrome, since waiting for microbiological confirmation would take too long.

The main task of a surveillance system is to detect sudden changes in incidence (i.e. outbreaks or epidemics). In such situations it becomes important that the system's sensitivity for detecting cases is high. This sensitivity may be the sum of several factors, such as the clinician's diagnostic accuracy, microbiological test methods, reporting propensity, etc. On the other hand, the specificity need not be so high, as it is of little consequence if a few cases too many are reported in an epidemic situation.

Such surveillance of incidence cannot be restricted to overall figures for a nation – it must also look at regional differences. An increased incidence in one part of a country may be masked by a decreased incidence somewhere else, keeping the total constant. In short, a surveillance system looks for clusters of disease in time and in space.

However, there is a need for a note of caution concerning surveillance data. Increasingly, such data are being used for purposes other than cluster alert. They are being utilized to monitor long-term trends, to make international comparisons, and to analyse the costs and benefits of preventive measures. Such uses put quite new demands on the quality of the data, and on the stringency of the epidemiological analysis. This has given national and regional surveillance units in several countries a new role, having to switch from outbreak investigations to more subtle analyses – a change with which some of them are still trying to come to terms.

CASE DEFINITIONS

From the original demands for high sensitivity to detect outbreaks and clusters to the growing current demands for correctness of data (i.e. high specificity), surveillance systems have a problem with case definitions. For most diseases it is impossible to design a case definition that is both wide and correct at the same time. As was pointed out in Chapter 8, the PPV and NPV of a given case definition will also vary with the incidence of the disease under surveillance. Taking measles in a high-incidence and a low-incidence country as an example, a clinical case definition of fever, rash and cough will have a high PPV in the former, but a very low one in the latter. In a country with a high level of measles vaccination coverage, most of the cases that fulfil this case definition will probably be other viral infections or adverse drug reactions.

One way to solve this problem is to allow for different levels of case definition in a surveillance system. A common approach is to define 'possible', 'probable' and 'confirmed' cases with an increasing degree of specificity. A possible case is usually one which displays some clinical sign of the actual infection – or one for which information is incomplete. A probable case may be one which fulfils most of the clinical criteria and/or has an equivocal laboratory tests, and a confirmed case is one in which clinical and microbiological data confirm the diagnosis – or one with the correct clinical picture which is epidemiologically linked to another confirmed case. There is a curious tendency in people with a microbiological background to assume that 'confirmed' equals 'laboratory confirmed' – a view that completely overlooks the fact that the laboratory result is just one of the pieces in the jigsaw puzzle of infectious disease diagnosis.

Each case that is entered in the database should be labelled with its corresponding level of case definition, and this level should be maintained throughout the analysis. The end user of the data can then decide whether the wider or narrower net is most appropriate for his or her intended purpose.

DISCOVERING OUTBREAKS

There are no simple rules of thumb for deciding when an outbreak is under way. Just as with the word 'epidemic', definitions are difficult. For many diseases, such as salmonella, gonorrhoea or measles, there will be a steady trickle of notified cases, and the task is to detect when this endemic situation becomes replaced by an outbreak. Other diseases such as plague and rabies are sufficiently rare in Western countries to warrant an outbreak investigation after just one case.

Because for many diseases there will always be a number of expected cases reported each week, surveillance implies continuous comparison of the actual number of cases with the expected number. In a conscientious surveillance programme, even minor deviations should at least be noted and given a second thought, although this second thought may lead to the decision to do nothing. The question of what constitutes a minor deviation as opposed to an alerting one is very much a matter of experience, and in most national or regional surveillance units there will be written and unwritten standards for action. In all such units there will always have been instances of heightened vigilance in response to suspected outbreaks, which were subsequently disregarded and never reached public attention.

Even though the aim of a notification system is to give the central agency power to detect outbreaks, many outbreaks are in reality first detected by astute clinicians. The best recent example is the discovery of AIDS. In the summer of 1981 two groups of clinicians in the USA almost simultaneously reported an unexpected incidence of strange diseases in young homosexual men, characterized by pneumonia caused by *Pneumocystis carinii* in Los Angeles,[1] and the skin tumour Kaposi's sarcoma in New York[2]. The US Centers for Disease Control in Atlanta immediately reacted to those reports and started a surveillance scheme, which finally led to the description of the new disease, but the original observation was made by clinicians.

ANALYSING OUTBREAKS

Once an outbreak has been established, the normal 'passive' surveillance that relies on notifications is often replaced by a more active phase, in which investigators are sent to the affected area to collect more information, much as was described in the previous chapter. However, since a routine surveillance system is devised to detect changes in the incidence of a number of listed diseases, the specific cause is usually known for outbreaks noted at a central level, and the investigation will focus on possible sources.

The need to cover a wider geographical area is evident from, for example, the present food distribution patterns of most countries, where an infected foodstuff may be distributed over wide areas, and where sporadic cases may appear in many different places, without being recognized as parts of an outbreak. A good example of this is the contamination of chocolate bars with salmonella in the UK in the early 1980s.[3]

During May 1982, three cases of infection with *Salmonella napoli* were reported to the Communicable Disease Surveillance Centre. Because there had only been 15 cases diagnosed in the UK during the previous 30 years, this incidence was higher than expected. Calculated as a yearly incidence it would correspond to 36 cases, compared with the expected 0.5. A total of 29 additional cases were reported in June.

The investigation started with telephone interviews and visits to determine the date of onset, geographical distribution and age and sex of the patients. It became clear that most of the cases lived in south-east England, and that children below the age of 15 years represented the majority.

Quite early on, the investigators started to suspect a brand of imported chocolate bars. In early July, they performed a small case–control study in which they collected food histories for the week preceding the illness from 17 patients. In order to investigate exposures in an outbreak like this, it is very important that secondary cases – infected by someone else in the family – are not included. As was pointed out in the previous chapter, such cases may not have had the exposure one is trying to assess, and adding them will introduce a misclassification, which will weaken the strength of any association that is found. Therefore one has to be quite careful when ascertaining dates of onset, and one also requires a knowledge of the incubation times of salmonella infections.

A total of 24 controls were chosen by asking the patients or their parents to name a household in the neighbourhood with people in the same age groups, or just by randomly approaching a neighbouring house. The controls were asked about food consumption during the week preceding the illness in the corresponding case. Note the choice of time period here. In order to obtain adequate control data it would not be appropriate to ask the controls what they ate during the last week. They must be asked about exposures during exactly the same time period as that when the cases were presumably exposed.

The 2×2 table for this first case–control study appeared as follows:

	Ate chocolate bar	Did not eat chocolate bar	
Case	9	8	17
Neighbour	0	24	24
	9	32	41

Over half of the cases had eaten (or remembered that they had eaten) chocolate bars, compared with none of the controls. Since there is a zero in the lower left-hand cell, we cannot calculate an odds ratio (it would be infinite), but using Fisher's exact test we find that the probability that the cases and controls would have these patterns of chocolate consumption just by chance is less than 0.0001.

This investigation led to the recall of the chocolate bars from all shops from late July, but during July and the first half of August more cases were diagnosed, and extended collection of faecal samples also revealed a number of asymptomatic carriers.

In total, 58% of the cases were under 15 years of age, and 60% of the older cases were women. The geographical analysis showed that during the first few months, almost all of the cases came from south-east England, where the chocolate bars were first marketed, whereas during the latter half of the outbreak, most of the cases were from northern England, where sales started in late June. The final case–control study included 93 cases and 122 controls, and the 2×2 table was as follows:

	Ate chocolate bar	Did not eat chocolate bar	
Case	57	36	93
Neighbour	3	119	122
	60	155	215

The OR for chocolate bars was (57/36)/(3/119) = 62.8, with a 95% confidence interval from 18.5 to 213, which is comfortably above 1. Thus there seems to have been a strong association between disease and chocolate bar consumption.

A good example of the usefulness of international surveillance comes from outbreaks of Legionnaires' disease in holiday travellers from northern Europe staying in Mediterranean resorts. In several instances it has been shown that *Legionella* can be spread from hotel air-conditioning systems or showers, and some tourists will become ill on returning home. The number of cases detected in each country may be very small, but by combining data from the different home countries of tourists who stayed in the same hotel, it becomes possible to elucidate the cause of the outbreak and to instigate preventive measures.

VALIDITY OF NOTIFICATION DATA

The most important problem in the interpretation of notification data concerns their validity. Do they really measure what we want them to measure? Is the yearly number of notified cases of a certain disease equal to the incidence? Can observed changes over time be safely interpreted as representing changes in the underlying incidence?

The number of patients reported with a certain disease will be influenced by many factors that may well change over time or between different places, and this will create biases when comparisons are made. Some such factors are listed below:

Attendance patterns

People's propensity to seek medical care cannot be assumed to be constant. The distance to the nearest hospital or clinic will play a role, as will costs and waiting times. Media reports of an outbreak will always bring more people to the clinic, and a proportion of these will probably have milder infections which would not ordinarily have made them come. Public awareness will thus increase the observed incidence.

Diagnostic methods

New tests that make it possible to diagnose atypical or asymptomatic cases of a disease will obviously lead to an increased reported incidence. A rather nice example comes from the introduction of chlamydia cultures in Sweden in the late 1970s (see Figure 13.1).

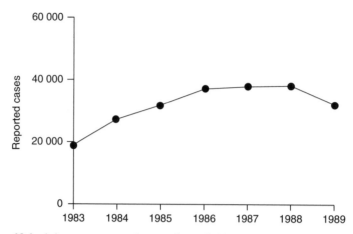

Figure 13.1 Laboratory-reported cases of genital chlamydia infection in Sweden during the period 1983–89.

There seemed to be a substantial increase in the incidence of chlamydia infections during the first part of the decade, with a doubling of cases between 1983 and 1987. However, what in fact happened was that more and more of the microbiological laboratories started to set up chlamydia testing and make it available to clinicians during this time. By plotting the total number of cultures performed each year we obtain the graph shown in Figure 13.2.

The second graph shows an almost perfect parallel increase in the numbers of samples taken and patients diagnosed between 1983 and 1986. Each year, one-tenth of the samples turned out positive. Therefore the apparent epidemic of chlamydia was most probably due to improved diagnostic facilities, and not to increased transmission. There is no reason to believe that there were fewer cases in 1980 than in 1987 – we just could not find them at

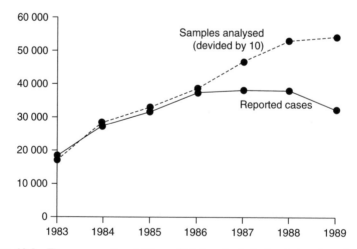

Figure 13.2 The same graph as in Figure 13.1, but also including the number of samples analysed each year (divided by 10 so that the scales are equal).

that time. (In addition, one can see that after 1988 the number of reported cases started to decrease although testing was still increasing, which supports the suspicion that there had been a real decrease in incidence after that time.)

Screening

A related problem concerns the setting up of screening programmes for asymptomatic infections. Such programmes will always lead to an apparent increase in incidence – 'Seek, and ye shall find.' However, this situation is quite far removed from the original surveillance model, in which sick people came to the doctor and were diagnosed.

In order to separate the cases found through screening from the symptomatic ones, notification forms now sometimes include a question about why the test was performed (patient's initiative, clinical suspicion, screening, etc.). In my experience it is often difficult for a doctor to specify this precisely. There may be several factors underlying the decision to perform a test, and the request to single out just one is often artificial.

Reporting propensity

Although many countries have statutory notification for a number of diseases, adherence to this legislation varies enormously between them. Comparison between countries of figures published in national statistics is for the most part meaningless unless one has reliable information on the completeness of notification behind those figures. In general, notification works better in countries with a nationalized health-care system than in countries with many independent clinics and laboratories.

Notification percentages may also vary within countries, and doctors often show similar behaviour to patients in that when there is increased media awareness of a certain disease, those cases become diagnosed and notified more readily.

Attendance patterns, diagnostic methods, screening and reporting propensity are all examples of biases (an appropriate term for this type of bias would be *assessment bias*) that could enter notification data, and they highlight the caution with which such data need to be approached. Does this mean that such surveillance systems fulfil no useful purpose? The answer is not necessarily, so long as one remembers their original *raison d'être*, which is to detect sudden changes in incidence for a number of listed diseases. To this end, it does not matter if only a proportion of all physicians report their cases, so long as this proportion remains roughly constant over time. For example, if a steady 15% of the doctors in a country are careful about sending in their notifications, incidence changes on a national scale will be detected anyway. Furthermore, the other sources of bias listed above will tend to be less problematic if the time scale is short.

There is another somewhat philosophical problem linked to the use of notification data to describe routes of transmission. Let us consider the example of infection with *Campylobacter pylori* and chicken consumption in Sweden. Not long after the bacterium was first described, it was found to be part of the normal intestinal flora of many birds. There were also some early reports of small family outbreaks of campylobacter diarrhoea after eating undergrilled chicken. The connection between chicken and this infection soon became well known to most clinicians, and they started asking their campylobacter patients if they had eaten chicken during the week or so before the onset of the illness. Chicken happens to be a very common food in Sweden, and a high proportion of the patients would answer 'yes', even though the chicken they ate might have had nothing to do with their disease. On the notification form, the clinician would put 'eaten chicken' in the box for possible risk factors. Thus a large number of the forms on campylobacter enteritis that were received by the national surveillance institute would state chicken as the most probable source, and in next year's annual report it would stand out as the most common risk factor. This would in turn further increase the clinicians' awareness of this route of infection, which would lead even more of them to ask about chicken consumption, and so on. This example points to the intrinsic 'conservative' nature of notification systems, especially if the risk comes from an exposure that is common, but which is only rarely the cause of disease. Most physicians will feel quite satisfied when their interview with the patient has revealed one established risk factor, and in situations such as this a notification system may tend to overestimate the importance of this factor and fail to detect other important routes of transmission.

NOTIFICATION DELAYS

There will always be a delay between diagnosis of a case and the arrival of the notification form at the central surveillance agency. This obviously has consequences for prevention, and you will find that the majority of reported point source outbreaks in the literature had actually subsided well before they were detected.

Reporting delays may also have statistical implications. Published surveillance statistics usually date cases by the day on which the form was received, not by the actual date of diagnosis or onset. Thus cases diagnosed late in one year may be registered the following year. For example, a curve showing weekly incidence over a period of 1 year may indicate low incidence during holiday periods (when there are fewer staff and everyone is too busy to fill in notification forms), and then a notable peak (when all of the forms were mailed at the same time). Such a peak could easily give a novice reader the mistaken impression that there had been a real epidemic just after the holiday period.

The issue of notification delays is quite important for surveillance, but it has not received much attention. One exception is a study from the UK in 1987[4], which used the information on notification slips to estimate the time from diagnosis to receipt of the form for 15 different diseases. Delay was found to vary according to both region and disease, being 5 days on average for measles but more than 2 months for tuberculosis. It also seemed to be increasing during the study period.

Another example is given in Figure 13.3, which shows the distribution of delays for all 30 733 notifications of campylobacter infection in Sweden during the years 1992 to 1998. The peak of registration of notifications at the Swedish Institute for Infectious Disease Control is 2 weeks after the onset of disease. After 3 weeks, 50% of the notifications have been made, but 10% of cases still remain unnotified 45 days after the onset of disease.

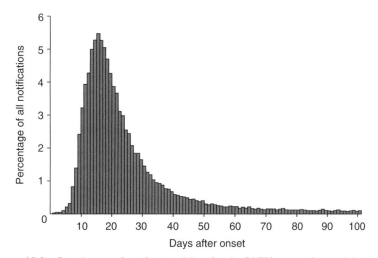

Figure 13.3 Distribution of notification delays for the 30 733 cases of campylobacter infection reported in Sweden during the period 1992–98. (Analysis courtesy of Johan Lindbäck, SMI.)

However, it was not until the emergence of the AIDS epidemic that a more systematic study of notification delays began. Accurate knowledge of past incidence is critical for projections of the future size of the epidemic. First, it was found in several Western countries that around 10–20% of all cases were never notified. Secondly, even for notified cases there were often long delays, so that typically only 80% of cases were reported in the year of diagnosis, and some cases were still being reported 2 or more years after they had first been diagnosed. The pattern of this reporting delay has been studied in several countries, and it has to be corrected for in models of future AIDS incidence. Similar problems now apply to the interpretation of data on variant Creutzfeldt–Jakob's disease, where the time of diagnosis is uncertain for several cases, and is sometimes changed retrospectively. The epidemic is thus described in terms of year of death, but even this reporting contains delays.

The increasing use of electronic notification of findings directly from the microbiological laboratory to the surveillance centre reduces delays considerably. Such reports usually contain very little epidemiological information, but if the name of the doctor requesting the test is included, it will be possible to contact him or her directly in order to obtain for a fuller picture.

FEEDBACK OF INFORMATION

Probably the most important part of a surveillance system that builds on the active participation of a large number of physicians is information feedback. If the central agency collects the data and analyses it, but fails to report back relevant findings to the people working in the field, their interest in reporting will wane. They must feel that the information they receive in return for spending time filling in forms is relevant to them in their daily work with patients. Adequate and timely information could aid them in making diagnoses and choosing treatments, and also in increasing vigilance with regard to specific diseases.

You will find solemn declarations like the above paragraph in any text on surveillance, but proper feedback is a difficult task. In most epidemic situations it has to be rapid, because it is of little use being told about an epidemic that has already subsided. It must also be clinically relevant, which is why it is important that the people responsible for the dissemination of the collated information keep in constant contact with the physicians who are the recipients.

The Internet has facilitated feedback considerably, and many national surveillance centres now display their data publicly almost as soon as they have been checked and corrected. The problem is now becoming more one of trying to supply the periphery with only the relevant information, and not drowning practitioners with undigested floods of data.

SENTINEL SYSTEMS

A sentinel system should ideally build on a random sample of the general practitioners in the country in question. This is seldom achievable, since reporting takes time, and many doctors may not have any special interest in mild to moderate infections. One therefore tries to obtain as good a geographical spread as possible by including interested colleagues. The average density of sentinel doctors in various European systems is usually around 1 per 30 000 to 100 000 members of the population.

Sentinel systems generally only report weekly number of patients with a certain disease (e.g. gastroenteritis or influenza-like illness), with little or no information about each case. Thus they only inform us about changes in overall incidence. Since they are based solely on clinical diagnosis, sensitivity is often very good, but specificity may be low.

In order to compare data between doctors and over time, some type of denominator must be used. This is often the number of patients on the doctor's list, or the population of the surrounding area, but it has been shown that the total number of patients seen during the reporting week is often a better denominator. This denominator takes into account holidays, absence because of meetings, and other events that may disturb the regular weekly pattern.

OTHER DATA SOURCES

Active surveillance cannot rely solely on notifications – it must make use of all of the available sources. These include laboratory reports, informal contacts with colleagues, media items, and sometimes even rumours. Often a more active role must be assumed, where clinicians are approached directly and asked about suspect cases. In a study of such a serious disease as paralytic poliomyelitis in England, only nine out of 19 cases that were finally analysed had been notified, the others were found by using other routes[5]. Obviously, however, the more one departs from a standardized data collection scheme, the less certain can one be that the data are representative.

SUMMARY

Surveillance is an important part of practical infectious disease epidemiology. It builds on the notion that whilst any one physician may only see one or two cases of an epidemic, and thus be unaware of it, the collected notifications at a regional or national level will make it possible to see the whole picture.

Active co-operation is required between clinicians and some central surveillance agency, where both parties should benefit from the activity. Rapid dissemination of analysed data back to the original suppliers in a form that they will find useful in their daily work is the most important component. A system in which the periphery feeds data into the centre without seeing any practical result is bound to falter.

REFERENCES

1. Centers for Disease Control. *Pneumocystis pneumonia* – Los Angeles. *Morb Mort Weekly Rep* 1981; **30**: 250–52.
2. Centers for Disease Control. Kaposi's sarcoma and pneumocystis pneumonia among homosexual men – New York City and California. *Morb Mort Weekly Rep* 1981; **30**: 305–8.
3. Gill ON, Bartlett CLR, Sockett PN *et al.* Outbreak of *Salmonella napoli* infection caused by contaminated chocolate bars. *Lancet* 1983; **1**: 574–7.
4. Clarkson JA, Fine PEM. Delays in notification of infectious disease. *Health Trends* 1987; **19**: 9–11.
5. Joyce R, Wood D, Brown D, Begg N. Paralytic poliomyelitis in England and Wales, 1985–91. *BMJ* 1992; **305**: 79–82.

Chapter 14
Measuring infectivity

Here we study how to answer probably the most commonly asked question about infectious diseases: 'How infectious is it?'. Different definitions of attack rate are discussed, with some published examples of studies. The importance of dose and immunity is exemplified, and the subclinical infections are mentioned.

One of the most important objectives of infectious disease epidemiology is obviously to measure infectivity. This is often quite difficult. One problem is that the meaning of the term is not well defined in most instances. Another is that infectivity may vary with different external factors. For example, it may be quite different in different types of contacts between an infectious individual and a susceptible one, as was pointed out in Chapter 11. A third problem when measuring the infectivity of a disease that is spread from person to person is trying to be certain that one person was infectious and the other was susceptible at the time of their contact.

Part of the semantic problem arises from lack of reflection on the concept of 'risk of becoming infected'. My risk of contracting influenza during the next epidemic season depends on three different factors:

1. the probability that I meet someone who is infectious with influenza. This probability depends on overall prevalence as well as on my contact pattern with other people;

2. the risk that the virus is transmitted when I meet someone who is infectious. This risk in turn depends on how close our contact is;

3. the probability that I am already immune to the strain responsible for the next epidemic.

Of these three factors, only the second is concerned with infectivity in the strict sense. However, any numerical value that is given for infectivity (or attack rate) will have to be accompanied by a definition of the type of contact to which it applies.

The basic assumption in all calculations of attack rates is that all of the people in the denominator were exposed to the pathogen. There is seldom any way of ascertaining this for certain, and it becomes a question of common sense and probabilities. For airborne infections it depends on proximity, wind direction and the volume of the space in which the index case and the exposed individual were congregated.

With foodborne infections it should be realized that the pathogen may not be evenly distributed within the food. A pie that has been infected with a few *Salmonella* bacteria and left at room temperature some time before it is to be consumed may show large variations in the number of bacteria per bite.

When studying the effect of condom usage on the risk of STI transmission, one must take several factors into account. Was the condom used throughout intercourse? Did it break? Could fingers have transferred the infection?

Earlier estimates of the risk of sexual transmission of the hepatitis C virus encountered the problem that a serological test for the disease could only show that a person had been infected once, not that they were still infectious, and different studies yielded conflicting results. The situation improves with the use of methods to detect viral RNA in patients, but even so the attack rate may vary with antigen level, and there is uncertainty about what happens below the detection threshold.

EXAMPLES – HOUSEHOLD INFECTIONS

One of the best studies of infectivity that has been performed was the one by Hope Simpson mentioned in Chapter 4. He wanted to measure the attack rates of measles, chicken-pox and mumps,[1] being well aware of the above problems. The design was as described below.

First he observed that 'the epidemic pattern depends in part on the natural characters of the parasite, [and] in part on the human host'. He went on to say that he wanted to eliminate any disturbing influence of human behaviour on his measurements, or in modern epidemiological jargon he stated that: he wanted to control for differences in contact patterns. He achieved this by looking only at transmission within households. The study was undertaken in an area of Gloucestershire between 1947 and 1951, and aimed to collect data on all exposures and transmissions of these three diseases in households in the area. The assumption that Hope Simpson made is obviously that the contact pattern – and thus the risk of exposure to a case – was sufficiently similar in all of the families to justify the calculation of average values across households.

The exact method of ascertaining the index cases is not described in his article, and one must assume that these cases were the children who were diagnosed by the local general practitioners. After a case had been diagnosed, a member of the epidemiological research unit visited this household several times to check up on the contacts. This method should be described as active surveillance, where cases are actually sought and not just routinely reported. The parents were also carefully asked whether any of the other children had had this disease before.

All susceptible siblings then constituted a cohort in which the risk of disease after contact with an index case could be calculated. The members of this cohort entered the study at different dates during a 4-year period, but since the risk of transmission should be the same in 1947 as in 1951, each sibling's time in the study can be regarded as starting on the day when the index case became ill.

A general problem with studies of transmission in households concerns the counting of the number of exposures. In families with only two children it is easy, as the sibling who is not the primary case is only exposed once. However, if there are three or more children, matters can become complicated. Suppose there are five children in a family – Adam, Beatrice, Cecil, David and Eusophryne. Adam is a primary case, and he infects Beatrice, but Cecil, David and Eusophryne escape the first round. Then Beatrice infects Cecil, but David and Eusophryne still remain susceptible. Thus in this family there were two transmissions, but what is the number of exposures? One way of counting them would be to list the number of susceptible individuals exposed to every new generation of cases as shown in Figure 14.1.

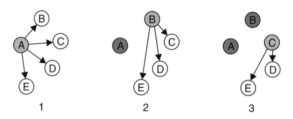

Figure 14.1 Three generations of exposures and transmission of an infection in a family with five children. White circles denote susceptible individuals, grey circles denote infectious individuals and black circles denote immune individuals. Arrows denote exposures.

Adam exposes four susceptible individuals, and then becomes immune. In the second generation, Beatrice exposes three susceptibles, and in the third generation, Cecil only exposes two susceptible individuals, since Adam and Beatrice are already immune. In this example there would thus be nine exposures of susceptible individuals in total.

This method of counting every new round of exposures due to the secondary, tertiary, etc. cases in the family gives a figure for the attack rate that Hope Simpson calls the 'susceptible exposure attack rate'. It is a very well-defined measure of infectivity, but is sometimes quite difficult to obtain. An alternative measure is called the 'household secondary attack rate', where all non-primary cases in a household are pooled together in the calculation. In the above example, the household attack rate would be 50%, since two out of four siblings were infected. The susceptible exposure attack rate according to Hope Simpson would be only 2/9, or 22%. You can see that it becomes crucial exactly how one defines the measure of attack rate. In order to calculate the susceptible exposure attack rate, it is also very important to sort out the generations of cases.

For both types of measures of attack rate, there may be a problem with the true number of susceptible individuals: whereas subclinical cases of measles are rare, chicken-pox can sometimes be very discrete, and a mumps infection can be quite asymptomatic. Some children may thus have been regarded as susceptible who were in fact immune. The figure we are looking for is the number of transmissions divided by the number of susceptible children exposed, but if exposures of immune children are entered into the denominator, then the calculated attack rate will be too low. The problem will be worse for the susceptible exposure attack rate method, since counting such exposures twice will increase the magnitude of this error.

Another problem concerns how multiple exposures should be accounted for. If there are two simultaneous primary cases in the household, how many exposures do the siblings receive?

Hope Simpson carefully emphasizes that his estimates of attack rates only apply to spread within families, and that other studies must be performed to assess attack rates in other settings. One might add that the figures only strictly apply to families of the sizes and living conditions that were prevalent in western England around 1950.

A rather similar study of household attack rates was performed in the USA in the late 1970s.[2] The aim was to measure the risk of household spread of invasive *Haemophilus influenzae* (HI) infections.

The index cases were patients with HI meningitis reported to the state health departments in 20 American states during an 18-month period. In total, 1403 such patients had their infections confirmed by culture of blood or cerebrospinal fluid (CSF). The families of 1147 of these patients were then investigated by the state or local health department, which assessed the number of actual contacts in each household and followed them for 30 days after the index case became ill. Secondary household cases were again confirmed by isolation of HI from blood or CSF. In total, there were 4311 household contacts, of whom 1687 were less than 6 years of age.

This study is also an example of a cohort design, in which all exposed family members are followed in order to assess the risk of infection. Each family enters the cohort on the day when the index case becomes ill, and remains in the study for 30 days, and the analysis is performed as if all families entered the study simultaneously. The study might have been prospective (if index cases were reported quickly, and the health department visited the families immediately) or retrospective (if there was a delay in reporting, and the 30 days had already passed when the health department staff came around). It is also an example of passive surveillance to find the index cases, and of active surveillance to find the secondary cases.

Nine associated cases of serious HI infection in eight households occurred within 30 days after the onset of meningitis in the index case. The risk of transmission was calculated according to the age of the susceptible subject (see Table 14.1).

Table 14.1 Household attack rate of *Haemophilus influenza* infection by age in a study from the USA (*Source:* Ward et al.[2])

Age (years)	Number at risk	Number ill	Risk (%)	95% Confidence interval
<1	50	3	6.0	1.3–16.6
1	69	1	1.4	0.04–7.8
2–3	259	4	1.5	0.4–4.0
4–5	1309	1	0.1	0.002–0.4
6–9	607	0	0	0–0.6
10–19	431	0	0	0–0.9
≥ 20	1586	0	0	0–0.2
Total	4311	9	0.21	0.10–0.40

The confidence intervals for the strata with zero risk are calculated as described in Chapter 7 on the confidence interval of zero. If zero events are observed, the 'true' number could have been as high as 3.7. In the stratum 10–19 years, the upper limit for the 95% confidence interval is thus 3.7/431 = 0.9%. One can see that there was a marked difference in attack rates depending on age, with no cases appearing in contacts aged 6 years or older. This means that age would be an important confounder if one were to compare the attack rate of HI meningitis in two different populations.

In total, 70% of the associated cases occurred within 1 week of the index patient's disease, and the median serial interval for this type of infection should thus be less than 1 week. The incubation period might be longer if the primary cases were infectious for some time before they became ill.

This study gives a low estimate for the attack rate of serious HI infection, since index cases as well as contacts had to have a severe, laboratory-proven infection. Other forms of HI disease, such as pneumonia, cellulitis or otitis media might add to the risk of illness in household contacts, but they were not included. Since there was one family with two secondary cases (or one secondary and one tertiary case), the authors might have used the Hope Simpson definition of secondary attack rate in this household, but they only give the crude rates shown in the table above.

THE USE OF SUBTYPING

In the above study, the authors proceeded to use serotyping to show that all of the invasive infections in index and secondary cases were caused by HI type b, which is known to be more virulent than other HI strains.

This possibility of 'fingerprinting' the infectious agent is a nice feature of infectious disease epidemiology. If one thinks about it, it is really a continuous process that started with the discovery of bacteria in the last century. For example, it would be very difficult to study the epidemiology of diarrhoea without the tools to single out the different species that cause this condition.

The next step was the advent of serology about 80 years ago, which taught us to differentiate within species, thus increasing the potential to follow the path of a pathogen through the population. A good example is given by the subtyping of *Salmonella* species, which can help us to discover outbreaks and eliminate a source even if the overall incidence of salmonella infections is almost constant, just as was exemplified by the chocolate bar outbreak in the previous chapter.

The present leap concerns the different methods for 'genetic fingerprinting', which allow us to identify individual strains of bacteria or viruses by looking at specific sequences in their genomes. With techniques such as restriction fragment length polymorphism (RFLP), pulse-field gel electrophoresis (PFGE) and direct sequencing of the genome, it is often possible to chart the separate clones of microbes within a population where several sources of the same pathogen are operating simultaneously. Such genetic methods are often described by their proponents as a completely new and revolutionary tool for infectious disease epidemiology, but I tend to think of them as just another link in a long chain of methods for subtyping different pathogens. Much also remains to be elucidated concerning their applicability in real-life epidemiology, the most important aspect being measures of natural mutation speed for different species and in different situations. The two situations in which subtyping becomes important for calculating risks of transmission are as follows.

1. Did person A infect person B?

2. Can we find the same strain in our patient as in the suspect sample of food, water, etc.?

If the strains compared are genetically identical, then there is little problem (except if the resolution is too low or if the two pieces of nucleic acid compared are too short, so that there may still be differences in other parts of the genome). If they differ slightly, how big can this difference be and still permit us to say that they are from the same clone? To answer this question, we need to know how rapidly the pathogen mutates – in the first host until transmission, in the environment, and in the second host after infection. The full potential of genetic subtyping awaits very careful studies in which excellent epidemiological and laboratory work are combined.

OTHER EXAMPLES – SEXUALLY TRANSMITTED INFECTIONS

The sexual transmission of infections provides another field of study where the type of contact is sufficiently standardized to allow calculations of attack rates. As part of the previously cited study on chlamydia infection in Sweden, data from partner notification were utilized to calculate the risk of transmission of this bacterium.[3]

Almost 6000 young women were screened for chlamydia infection in a number of family planning clinics in Gothenburg. None of them had subjective symptoms of a genital infection, but 425 women were found to be culture positive for chlamydia. For 309 of these women it was possible to contact and test the male partner with whom they had last had intercourse before the diagnosis was made. In total 74 of these men, (24%), also had a chlamydia infection.

At first sight this looks like another nice cohort study, where 309 men were exposed to 309 women with chlamydia infection. We know that the women could not have become infected later, since this was their last intercourse before diagnosis. The attack rate of chlamydia infection would then be 24%. However, there are several difficulties involved in the interpretation of data such as these. First, we do not know who infected whom. Some of the infected men must have been the sources of the infections in the women, and were thus neither exposed nor susceptible. Secondly, some of the men could have been infected by another partner after their intercourse with an index woman. Thirdly, the median time between diagnosis of the index case and testing of the partner was 21 days, and for 10% of the men it was more than 2 months. Several men might have recovered from their infections – or had perhaps been taking antibiotics for other infections that cured their chlamydia infection as well. Fourthly, even if the figure of 24% was correct, it need not apply to the risk of transmission from an infected man to a susceptible woman.

Thus studies of the attack rate of STIs face several methodological problems, and many published studies are more like case reports where it has been possible to calculate the number of transmissions to partners of a single infectious individual.

As a rare example of the opposite situation, a rather elegant study of the risk of gonorrhoea transmission from females to males was conducted in the early 1970s on the crew members of a large US Navy vessel.[4] During passage from the American west coast across the Pacific Ocean, all sailors were tested for gonorrhoea infection, and those who were found to be infected were treated. The ship subsequently spent 4 days in an Asian port, during which time the crew had the opportunity to meet local prostitutes and barmaids. After leaving port, a sample of 537 men was again examined for gonorrhoea infection, and 54 men were now positive. Thus the overall attack rate was 10%, but that figure tells us nothing about transmission risk unless we also know the prevalence of infection in the women. This important piece of extra information was provided from the clinic that the registered prostitutes had to attend for bimonthly check-ups. In total, 511 of the approximately 8000 prostitutes in the area attended this clinic during the days when the ship was in port, and they were all examined for gonorrhoea. It was found that 90 of them were infected, with a prevalence of 17.6%.

The next step in the calculations requires two assumptions. The first is that the 511 women who were examined constituted a representative sample of all of the women the crew could have met. The second assumption is that the men chose women randomly with regard to infectious status – the women who were infected should not have a higher or lower probability of becoming a partner than the ones who were not infected. If these two assumptions hold, then 17.6% of the men would have been exposed to gonorrhoea, and since 10% became infected, the risk of transmission (i.e. attack rate) would be 10/17.6 = 57%.

Many models for the spread of STIs assume a constant attack rate per intercourse, and that the risk of transmission will increase with the number of episodes of intercourse that an infectious individual and a susceptible one have. (This is a good point at which to introduce a parenthesis about the calculation of risk in such situations. Let us assume that we are studying an STI for which there is some empirical evidence that the attack rate after one act of intercourse is 25%, and we want to calculate the risk of infection after having engaged in four acts of intercourse with an infectious partner. Someone who was unfamiliar with statistics might easily believe that this risk would be $4 \times 25 = 100\%$, but that is wrong. Risks cannot be added in this way, and the problem is somewhat similar to the discussion of risks and rates in Chapter 10. This is because the way of becoming infected in, say, the third intercourse is to escape infection in the first two, and then to become infected in the third. The probability of this event is less than 25%. The simplest way to estimate the total risk is as follows. First calculate the probability of *not* being infected at all during the four episodes of intercourse. This is equal to the chance of escaping infection the first time, which is 75%, multiplied by the chance of not being infected the second time, which is again 75%, and so on. The probability of not being infected after four acts of intercourse is thus $0.75 \times 0.75 \times 0.75 \times 0.75 = 0.32$. Then remember that the probability of something happening is 1 minus the probability that it does not happen, which means that the risk of *having* become infected is $1 - 0.32$, or 0.68. The risk is thus 68% after four acts of intercourse, and not 100%.)

In the above example involving gonorrhoea among the naval crew, the authors tried to use this formula to calculate the risk per act of sexual intercourse, since most of the men had had intercourse more than once with each partner. They obtained the unexplained finding that the attack rate per act of intercourse in the white sailors was 19%, but as high as 53% among black crew members. They suggested that one possible reason for this could be a selection bias among the women, in that the prostitutes whom the white men met might have had a lower prevalence of gonorrhoea.

We shall be examining more studies that measure attack rate in Chapter 19 on the epidemiology of vaccination.

DOSE

Another important aspect of infectivity concerns the dose of the pathogen that a susceptible person receives. You should note that there is a close connection between the concept of 'dose' and the concept of 'type of contact' discussed previously. A closer contact between an infectious individual and a susceptible one will probably lead to the transmission of a higher dose.

In most real-life situations it becomes almost impossible to measure the infective dose, which is counted as the number of bacteria or viruses. How do we know exactly how many virus particles a measles case spreads when he or she is coughing? How many of these must enter a susceptible individual in order to cause infection and/or disease? We know that the blood of an acute case of hepatitis B may contain up to 10^9 virus particles/mL, but in the study of percutaneous accidental transmission in hospital, how do we know the exact volume of blood that is inoculated into a susceptible person?

For enteric infections, the relationship between dose and risk of infection has been studied quite thoroughly in regular trials. Several such trials took place in the USA in the 1950s and 1960s, using prisoner volunteers as subjects.

In one such experiment,[5] controlled doses of *Salmonella bareilly* were given to three groups of six volunteers. Table 14.2 shows the results.

Table14.2   Attack rate as a function of ingested dose of bacteria (*Source*: McCollough and Eisle[5])

Dose	Ill	Healthy	Attack rate
125 000	1	5	17
695 000	2	4	33
1 700 000	4	2	67

The attack rate clearly increases with dose, and it seems that a dose of around 1 000 000 bacteria will cause disease in half of the subjects exposed to it. This figure is sometimes called ID_{50} (i.e. the dose of a pathogen that will cause disease in 50% of exposed susceptible subjects). A possible source of error in calculations such as these is that some of the ill subjects were not infected in the experiment, but that they became secondary cases to some real primary case. However, the authors assure the reader that this could not have happened. One should also note that the number of subjects involved in the study was small, and therefore the confidence intervals for the attack rates will be very wide (for the estimate 33% in the middle line in the table the 95% confidence interval will be from −5 to 71%, using the formula for a proportion given in Chapter 7).

In this definition of attack rate, only clinical cases were counted. Changes in agglutination titres (a serological and rather crude test for salmonella infection) were also measured in all subjects, but only showed any increase in four of the seven cases. However, the number of days for which the subjects excreted *Salmonella* in faeces are shown in Figure 14.2 below.

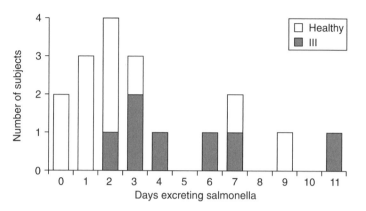

Figure 14.2   Number of days on which salmonella could be found in stools in 18 volunteers given controlled doses of *Salmonella bareilly*. (*Source*: McCollough and Eisele[5].)

Thus two of the subjects only excreted *Salmonella* on the day of the trial, three of them continued to excrete *Salmonella* during the next day, but not for longer, and so on. Most of the subjects who did not become ill thus excreted the bacteria for only a day or two, and these may have been just those bacteria that they had ingested. However, the two healthy subjects who excreted *Salmonella* for 7 and 9 days, respectively, probably had subclinical infections. They were both given the medium dose.

This example once again demonstrates the importance of the case definition in calculating attack rates. When reading studies on attack rates or on infectivity, one should always check whether or not subclinical cases were included, and how they were ascertained.

In a similar study of typhoid,[6] volunteers received controlled doses of *Salmonella typhii* with 10^6-fold variation in the number of bacteria given (Table 14.3).

In this example, too, the ID_{50} seems to be around 1 000 000 bacteria, and the higher numbers of subjects in each group give better confidence intervals for the attack rates than in the previous example.

Table 14.3   Attack rate of *Salmonella typhii* infection with increasing doses of bacteria ingested (*Source*: Hornick et al.[6])

Dose	III	Healthy	Attack rate (%)
10^3	0	14	0
10^6	32	84	28
10^7	16	16	50
10^8	8	1	89
10^9	40	2	95

Another example of experimental infection comes from a study of gonorrhoea in male volunteers in the USA in the early 1990s.[7] A controlled dose of gonococci, ranging from 10^4–10^6 bacteria, was instilled with a catheter in the urethra of 47 men. Gonococcal infection developed in 27 individuals. The higher dose led to infection in 9 out of 10 men, and the lower dose to infection in 6 out of 10 men. The higher dose also led to a shorter incubation time.

In some outbreaks it has been possible to obtain an estimate of the infective dose in 'real-life' situations. For bacterial enteric infections this becomes possible if some part of the infected food item remains and can be tested after the outbreak has been discovered. One example comes from an outbreak of *Salmonella eastbourne* in North America in 1974.[8]

This outbreak was spread over several states in the USA and Canada, and it was discovered by the US national surveillance programme. Shortly after the detection of the outbreak, a telephone-based case–control study was undertaken which involved interviewing 28 cases in different states. Only primary cases in each family were interviewed, and each family was asked to name two controls. The odds ratio for having eaten a certain brand of Christmas-wrapped chocolate balls was 9, with a narrow confidence interval. Several families still had chocolate balls at home, and samples for salmonella infection were taken from these balls. The mean number of bacteria was 2.5 per gram. The investigators assumed that a typical case would have eaten one pound of chocolate, giving a total dose of 1000 bacteria – much lower than in the above experiment.

Several other studies have shown lower doses in outbreaks from food or water than in the controlled experiments described above. There is obviously always a problem in demonstrating that the density of bacteria remaining several days to weeks after the exposure is the same as it was originally. This can sometimes be assessed by controlled contamination of similar food, which is then subjected to the same process (freezing, etc.) as the source of the outbreak. However, chocolate is a particularly good medium in this respect, since *Salmonella* bacteria are stable in chocolate – they neither die nor multiply.

Thus numerical calculations of infective doses can sometimes be made for enteric infections, where the number of infecting organisms can be measured or estimated. For most other infections, and especially for those that are spread by contact or via the air, this is generally impossible. When estimating the relationship between dose and attack rate for such infections, one will therefore have to use closeness of contact as a proxy measure for dose, assuming that a susceptible individual who is near to a case for a long time will be exposed to a higher dose than a casual contact of the same case.

We have already seen one instance of different attack rates for different types of contacts in the monkey-pox example described in Chapter 4. A similar study was conducted during an outbreak of smallpox in a village in Dahomey in 1967.[9]

The disease was introduced into the village (with some 300 inhabitants) by a woman and her two children, who all developed smallpox around the time of their arrival. The disease spread to eight other households over a period of two and a half months. Six of these households were immediate neighbours.

The household attack rate in the nine afflicted houses was 17 cases out of 34 exposed, or 50%. The number of transmissions to someone outside the household was 7, and based on a denominator of around 270 (since 34 of all the people in the village were household contacts), the attack rate between households would be around 3%. This indicates that close and prolonged contact is usually necessary for spread, and it is difficult to think of any explanation for this other than a correlation between risk of infection and dose.

Another example of increasing attack rate with closer contact comes from an episode in which multi-drug-resistant tuberculosis (MDR-TB) appears to have spread during a transcontinental flight.[10] In May 1994, a passenger with undiagnosed open TB flew from Chicago to Honolulu. Soon afterwards the diagnosis was made, and the passengers and crew were notified of their potential exposure, advised to have a skin test, and asked to complete a questionnaire. In total, 15 people who had been on the plane had positive tuberculin skin tests, but nine of these had other risk factors for TB. It was thus assumed that six fellow travellers had Mantoux-converted after exposure to the index patient. They had all been seated in the same section of the aircraft as the index case.

The investigators had managed to reach 68 (the six cases above plus 62 others) of the passengers who had had seats in this section, and they were divided into those sitting within two rows of the index patient and those sitting further away. The attack rates were calculated to be $4/13 = 30.8\%$ for those sitting close to the index case, and $2/55 = 3.6\%$ for those who were more distant ($P = 0.01$), which supports the view that attack rate increases with proximity and thus with dose.

IMMUNITY

This problem was touched upon earlier with regard to the Hope Simpson data. Immune individuals should not be entered among the susceptible subjects exposed. It is often impossible to know whether a person was immune when they were exposed, and even if serology could be performed after the exposure, one may not always be able to distinguish between a previous immunity and a subclinical infection due to the exposure.

One nice example of the opposite situation concerns a measles outbreak that occurred in a dormitory at a US university in 1985.[11]

Between 31 January and 7 February the Red Cross held a blood drive at the university, during which students were asked to donate blood. Almost simultaneously, a measles outbreak started there, the first case being diagnosed on 28 January, and the last on 20 March. Many of the students would thus have had blood samples taken just before the outbreak started. In total, 139 students living in the dormitory had donated blood, of whom 90 agreed to take part in a study, the aim of which was to analyse the association between antibody titres before exposure and subsequent risk of measles.

A measles case was defined as an illness characterized by a generalized maculopapular rash lasting for more than 3 days, fever greater than 38.3°C if measured, and at least one of the following: cough, coryza or conjunctivitis. Cases were confirmed by blood samples showing a fourfold or higher rise in antibody titre from the acute sample to the convalescent sample (see Chapter 16 for a discussion of antibody titres). One student developed a rash just 3 days after donating blood, and was excluded, since his antibody titre at the time of donation might already have been increasing.

Donated blood is usually kept in plastic bags, but there is always some blood left in the plastic tube leading into the bag (the 'pigtail'), and this could be collected for 80 of the 90 subjects in the study. Eight of the 90 donors had an illness that met the criteria of the clinical case definition, and measles was confirmed serologically in seven of these donors (post-illness serum was unavailable for one of them). If a pre-exposure antibody titre value of 1/120 was chosen as the cut-off value, the outcome was as follows:

	Antibody titre ≤ 1/120	Antibody titre > 1/120	
Measles	8	0	8
No measles	1	71	72
	9	71	80

The difference is highly significant ($P < 0.001$ by Fisher's exact test), and we can see that just one person with a low titre escaped infection. This is therefore a very nice example of how immunity influences attack rate in an outbreak.

It is difficult to think of any biases or confounders that could have distorted this finding. The students who volunteered for the study hardly had any knowledge of their pre-exposure titres, and all of the blood tests were performed blind to the case status of the students.

One possibility would be that the antibody measured had nothing to do with protection, but rather it was a marker for some real protective factor, but then the correlation between this confounder and titre must have been very high. The investigators could also demonstrate a rise in antibody titre in a number of students who did not develop measles, and we shall return to those results in a later chapter.

Modern research is also starting to reveal a quite new type of 'immunity' which has nothing to do with the immunity conferred by past infection or by vaccination. Some individuals seem to be genetically protected from infection with certain pathogens, since they apparently lack the cell-surface receptors necessary for the microbe to adhere to the human cell or to enter it. People who are homozygotic for the absence of the chemokine cell-surface receptor CCR5 seem to be resistant to infection by HIV. The finding that all cases of variant CJD tested so far are homozygotic for the amino acid methionine at codon 129 of the prion protein gene has led to speculation that people who are either homozygotic for valine at this site, or who are heterozygotic, may be immune to the disease. More findings of 'genetic immunity' such as these will of course influence how attack rates are perceived and calculated in the future.

OTHER COFACTORS

This chapter makes no attempt to list all of the factors that influence risk of infection. One often-mentioned example is the increased risk of enteric infections, especially cholera, in patients who suffer from achlorhydria of the stomach. The very low pH of the ventricle is an important defence mechanism against several infections.

We shall look at a somewhat unusual study that attempted to relate the degree of psychological stress to the infection rate from common cold viruses.[12]

The study was performed at the British Medical Research Council's Common Cold Unit in Salisbury – an institution that has produced several interesting findings on the epidemiology of common colds. The subjects were 154 men and 266 women volunteers aged 18 to 54 years. During the first 2 days the subjects underwent a thorough medical examination and answered three different questionnaires designed to measure their present degree of psychological stress. Subsequently, a solution containing either one of five different viruses or a saline placebo was dropped into each subject's nose, and they were then put in quarantine and monitored for infection and clinical symptoms.

The occurrence of infection was established using both virological and serological criteria. Clinical cold was established by subjects' reports and by clinical examination.

The results were analysed by logistic regression, where the outcome measure was either laboratory-verified infection or clinical cold. The explanatory factor was the degree of psychological stress as scored by the responses to the questionnaires. For both outcomes there was a significant increase in attack rate with increasing stress score. The rate of infection ranged from 74% to 90% and the incidence of clinical cold ranged from 27% to 47% going from the lowest to the highest stress value. These findings remained significant even after controlling for a number of confounders, such as age, allergic status, season, and virus-specific antibody status at baseline. Simply dividing the subjects into those with high stress vs. those with low stress gave an adjusted OR for infection of 5.8 and for illness of 2.2. The associations were similar for all five strains of virus tested. This study probably supports the popular belief that one becomes more susceptible to infection when one is feeling stressed.

SUBCLINICAL INFECTIONS

As I have mentioned several times now, the value of an attack rate very much depends on how a 'case' is defined. In many studies, the numerator only includes the cases that were diagnosed clinically. However, most people would probably want to include subclinical infections as well, especially if those patients can spread the disease further in the population. If such cases are to be detected, one needs serology, and in some instances one needs a sample that was taken before the exposure for comparison. This happened to be the case in the measles example above, but is generally quite a rare event.

(It should be noted that measles is one of the best diseases available for studying transmission, which has always made it a favourite with infectious disease epidemiologists. The attack rate is high, there are very few subclinical cases, the incubation time is short, and immunity after infection is lifelong. There are not many other infections for which these four statements are true. For example, in HIV infection the opposite of each statement applies.)

SUMMARY

Infectivity must be distinguished from 'risk of becoming infected', since this risk will also depend on the prevalence of infectious sources in the environment (e.g. mosquitoes, people, etc.).

It is unclear why not all susceptible individuals become infected when exposed. The dose of the pathogen is one important factor, but even with identical doses some people are infected and others are not. Perhaps there are temporary fluctuations in some type of non-specific immunological resistance, but if so they would be very difficult to study. In the absence of a precise biological understanding of the factors that govern infection in every single case, we resort to talking about the probability, or risk, of disease after a certain type of exposure. We call this measure the attack rate.

The relationship between attack rate and dose can be studied in cohort studies, both by ingestion of a known number of bacteria and in natural situations, when the dose encountered can be estimated afterwards. For diseases that are spread from person to person, closeness and duration of contact between an infectious individual and a susceptible one are often taken as proxy measures of the dose transmitted.

When measuring attack rates for diseases that are spread from person to person, careful elucidation of transmission routes and generations is essential. Several definitions of attack rate in such situations exist, and the susceptible exposure attack rate is probably the best defined and the one which most reliably measures infectivity. However, it is very sensitive to the erroneous inclusion of already immune subjects as exposed susceptibles.

REFERENCES

1. Hope Simpson RE. Infectiousness of communicable diseases in the household (measles, chicken-pox and mumps). *Lancet* 1952; **2**: 549–54.

2. Ward JI, Fraser DW, Baraff U, Plikaytis BD. *Hemophilus influenzae* meningitis. A national study of secondary spread in household contacts. *N Engl J Med* 1979: **301**: 122–6.

3. Ramstedt K, Forssman L, Giesecke J, Johannisson G. Epidemiological characteristics of two different populations of women with *Chlamydia trachomatis* infection and their male partners. *Sex Transm Dis* 1991; **18**: 46–51.

4. Hooper RR, Reynolds GH, Jones OG *et al.* Cohort study of venereal disease. I. The risk of gonorrhea transmission from infected women to men. *Am J Epidemiol* 1978; **108**: 136–45.

5. McCullough NB, Eisele CW. Experimental human salmonellosis. III. Pathogenicity of strains of *Salmonella newport, Salmonella derby* and *Salmomella bareilly* obtained from spray-dried whole egg. *J Infect Dis* 1951; **89**: 209–13.

6. Hornick RB, Greisman SE, Woodward TE, DuPont HL, Dawkins AT, Snyder MJ. Typhoid fever: pathogenesis and immunologic control. *N Engl J Med* 1970; **283**: 686–91.

7. Cohen MS, Cannon JG, Jerse AE *et al.* Human experimentation with *Neisseria gonorrhoeae:* rationale, methods and implications for the biology of infection and vaccine development. *J Infect Dis* 1994; **169**: 532–7.

8. Craven PC, Baine WB, Mackel DC *et al.* International outbreak of *Salmonella eastbourne* infection traced to contaminated chocolate. *Lancet* 1975; **1**: 788–92.

9. Henderson RH, Yekpe M. Smallpox transmission in Southern Dahomey. A study of a village outbreak. *Am J Epidemiol* 1969; **90**: 423–8.

10. Kenyon TA, Valway SE, Ihle WW, Onorato IM, Castro KG. Transmission of multidrug-resistant Mycobacterium tuberculosis during a long airplane flight. *N Engl J Med* 1996; **334**: 933–8.

11. Chen RT, Markowitz LE, Albrecht P *et al.* Measles antibody: re-evaluation of protective titers. *J Infect Dis* 1990; **162**: 1036–42.

12. Cohen S, Tyrell DAJ, Smith AP. Psychological stress and susceptibility to the common cold. *N Engl J Med* 1991; **325**: 606–12.

Chapter 15
Studying the natural history of infectious diseases

Here the epidemiological methods used to study the natural history of an infectious disease are touched upon, as well as the study of prognostic markers and cofactors for disease progression. Biases in such studies are discussed, and the importance of dose is once again exemplified.

This book deals more with the transmission, detection, diagnosis and prevention of infectious diseases than with their natural history and treatment. The reason for this is that the first four points are more particular to infectious disease epidemiology. Once a patient has become a case and starts developing the disease or is taken into hospital, the tools used for epidemiological study become similar for almost all groups of diseases.

Important questions about the natural history of an infectious disease include the following. What is the incubation time? What are the symptoms? How severe is the disease generally, and what are the risk factors for a more serious course of events? How long does the infection last? We have already encountered one such concept in Chapter 2, namely the case fatality rate, which measures how many of those who acquire an infection will die from it within some defined time period.

A closely related question concerns the effects of different drugs such as antibiotics and antiviral agents on the severity and outcome of a disease. Such questions are generally studied in regular clinical trials, with randomization, controlling and blinding. You will remember from Chapter 6 that the main conceptual difference between 'pure' epidemiological studies and clinical trials is that for the former we have to be content with the assignment of risk factors and subjects that nature provides, whereas for the latter we can choose subjects and assign exposures at will.

INCUBATION PERIODS

The easiest way to measure an incubation period is obviously in an outbreak situation, when a group of people have been exposed simultaneously. The epidemic curve of such an outbreak will give a good picture of the incubation time distribution, and if you remember the Legionnaires' disease outbreak example in Chapter 12, you may recall that the incubation time for this new disease was actually known before its aetiology was clarified. In more prolonged outbreaks, or when the infection is transmitted from person to person, one will need to interview cases carefully about when they could have been exposed. One of the nicest such studies performed is also one of the oldest. It concerns an outbreak of measles in the Faroe Islands, west of the coast of Norway, in 1846. At that time, these islands were part of Denmark, and the young Danish doctor Panum was sent by the authorities to investigate the outbreak.[1] In his report on the investigation, he points out that:

> The isolated situation of the villages, and their limited intercourse with each other, made it possible in many, in fact in most, cases to ascertain where and when the person who first fell ill had been exposed to the infection, and to prove that the contagion could not have affected him either before or after the day stated.

He interviewed a large number of cases, and seems to have followed the infection in almost every village of the islands, clarifying exactly who brought the infection to the village, and where he or she must have been infected. The clearest example relates to the village of Tjørnevig. On 4 June a boat with 10 men from Tjørnevig had gone to the village of Vestmannhavn to take part in a hunt for grind (a small whale). They spent part of the day in houses there, and Panum could later record that there had been measles cases in those houses during the days subsequent to the visit. On 18 June, exactly 14 days after the exposure, a measles rash developed in every one of the 10 men, after they had been feeling ill with cough and conjunctivitis for 2 to 4 days. Almost everyone else in Tjørnevig then developed a measles rash between 12 and 16 days later, except for a few who fell ill after a further 12 to 16 days.

From similar observations in other villages, Panum concluded that the incubation time from exposure to first symptoms of measles was 10 to 12 days, and to rash 14 days. The shortest serial interval was 12 days, showing that a case was infectious about 2 days before the rash developed.

He also made another observation concerning the natural history of measles, namely that the case fatality rate (CFR) increased with age. By making comparisons with average mortality from parish registers for the time period 1835 to 1845, he could show that during the period of the epidemic, overall mortality did not change at all in the 1–20 years age group, whilst in the 30–50 years age group it increased by a factor of 2.5, and for those aged 50–60 years it increased by a factor of 5.

Another finding, which has few parallels in infectious disease epidemiology, was factual data to support the theory that measles infection confers lifelong immunity. The previous measles epidemic on the Faroes had been 65 years earlier, in 1781, and since then the disease had been totally absent from the islands. Panum observed that not one person who had had measles in 1781 and who was still alive in 1846 had the disease a second time.

NATURAL HISTORY

The basic type of design for studying the natural history of an infectious disease is the cohort study. A cohort of patients who have been diagnosed with the disease are followed over time, and events and outcomes are recorded. In many such studies, a bias with regard to severity is introduced, which may or may not be a problem depending on one's point of view. Since they are generally based on patients diagnosed within the health-care system, and often on patients in hospital, such studies will tend to include patients whose disease is towards the more severe end of the scale, and asymptomatic or mild infections will not be diagnosed or included.

For several important diseases, the ratio of subclinical to clinical infections in an epidemic is very high. It has been estimated that for every apparent child with polio in an epidemic there are about 100 asymptomatic infected children in the population. Cholera is another disease in which many become infected but few become ill. In the absence of serology or bacterial culture, the normal natural history of such infections will not be properly understood.

If the results of a study of hospitalized patients are used to describe the natural history of a disease, the prognosis will seem worse than a general practitioner would find from his or her experiences, and even worse than a study that was based on all cases in the population. An infectious disease doctor may find that quite a high proportion of salmonella patients develop complications of the infection, such as arthritis or arteritis. However, since only a small proportion of salmonella infections are diagnosed, and an even smaller proportion are seen in hospital, the overall risk may not be very high.

On the other hand, if the aim of the study is not to describe the general natural history, but rather to inform hospital doctors about the complications they are likely to see, then such a study would not be biased – provided that the selection of patients is similar in the clinics where the findings of the study are read.

One example of a study that gives preliminary information on the natural history of a newly discovered disease comes from Venezuela.[2] In September 1989, an outbreak of a severe haemorrhagic disease was observed by physicians in Guanarito. It was first believed to be dengue, but one year later a new virus was isolated from a fatal case, and a serological test for this new Guanarito virus was developed from mouse ascitic fluid.

Between September 1990 and April 1991, 14 patients treated in a hospital in Guanare were diagnosed as being infected with this virus, either by isolation or by seroconversion.

The age range of the patients was 6–54 years, with most of the cases occurring in young adults, and they had been ill between 3 and 12 days before admission. The main presenting symptoms were fever, prostration, arthralgia and headache, and 13 of the 14 patients had one or more haemorrhagic manifestations. Nine of the 14 patients died within 1 to 6 days after admission.

The case fatality rate in this study was 9/14 = 0.64, but the sample is small. Let us use our formula for confidence intervals for a proportion from Chapter 7 to calculate a 95% confidence interval. The standard error of this proportion will be as follows:

$$\sqrt{\frac{0.64 \times 0.36}{14}} = 0.128$$

and the 95% confidence interval is given by 0.64 ± 1.96 × 0.128, which means that the CFR for this disease would be between 39% and 89%. The confidence interval becomes wide when the sample is small.

A more serious objection to the figure for the CFR concerns the selection of subjects. The authors remark that their case fatality rate is higher than reported for Lassa fever or Argentine haemorrhagic fever, but also that early studies of these diseases found very high rates, which were later modified when milder cases were diagnosed. They thus undertook a small seroepidemiological study of 57 family contacts of the cases and found six of these to have antibody to Guanarito virus, which supports the notion that the patients seen in the hospital had a more severe form of the disease.

A similar line of reasoning is expressed in a posting on ProMED (see Chapter 21) by C. Calisher on 1 February 2001 (Gulu was the epicentre of this Ebola outbreak in Uganda):

According to the latest figures (31 Jan 2001), there have been 428 cases, including 173 (40%) deaths for all of Uganda. In Gulu district there were 396 cases, including 150 deaths (38%), leaving 32 cases, including 23 deaths (72%), in Masindi and Mbarara districts. This suggests to me that only the most severe cases, most leading to death, have been detected outside Gulu district. If so, it follows that there might have been more cases, those less severe and undetected, outside Gulu district.

LATE SEQUELAE

Research interest is increasingly being focused on late or very late sequelae of acute infections. Much interest has focused – without any clear result – on the association between measles in childhood and multiple sclerosis much later in life. Another example, for which there is much more substantial support, is the association between infection with human papilloma virus and cervical cancer. If there is no reliable, long-lasting biological marker of past infection, a cohort design is usually necessary to study such late effects, since most people will not be able to recall an acute infection from 10 or 20 years ago. This means that good population-based registers are often needed.

One such study was performed to study the risk of Guillain–Barré syndrome after acute campylobacter enteritis in Sweden.[3] The Guillain-Barré syndrome (GBS) is a rapidly progressing, ascending paralysis which may become fatal without artificial ventilation. Its pathological mechanism is unknown, but it usually subsides after several months. An earlier case–control study had indicated that serological markers of recent campylobacter infection were more common in cases than in controls.

The study began by using the national hospital discharge registry to determine the annual incidence of GBS in the Swedish population during the 1990s. This figure was 1.8 cases per 100 000 members of the population, and it remained rather constant over the time period. The next step was to list the personal identifier numbers for all reported cases of campylobacter enteritis notified to the Swedish Institute for Infectious Disease Control during the time period 1987 to 1995. The total number of cases was 29 563. This list of patients was again compared with the hospital discharge registry to find out if any of them had been diagnosed with GBS in the 2-month period after their acute infection. Nine cases were detected, or 30.4 per 100 000 (95% CI: 13.9–57.8). The expected incidence over this 2-month period would have been the above 1.8 cases divided by 6, or 0.3 per 100 000. Thus from this study, based on two national registers, the risk of GBS after an acute campylobacter infection could be calculated to be around 100 times higher than in the general population.

PROGNOSTIC FACTORS

Similar cohort strategies can also be used to study individual patients with a certain disease factors that will be associated with outcome. An example of the basic structure of such studies is given by an investigation of the association between size of vegetation and outcome in infectious endocarditis in the USA.[4]

This study focused on right-sided endocarditis in intravenous drug users. It was performed as a retrospective cohort study in which the medical records of 121 such patients with 132 episodes of active endocarditis were reviewed. They had been treated in the Beth Israel Medical Center once or more between 1978 and 1986, and the inclusion criteria were right-sided valvular vegetation documented by two-dimensional echocardiography, history of intravenous drug use, two or more positive blood cultures, and at least two clinical signs compatible with active endocarditis (fever, septic emboli, heart murmur).

The authors used only two endpoints, namely death or discharge without any clinical signs of active endocarditis. In 30 of the 132 episodes the patients left the hospital before completion of treatment, and these were not included in the analysis. Of the remaining 102 episodes, 10 episodes ended with the patient's death, and 92 episodes were successfully treated. Three of the patients who died had complications other than a right-sided vegetation, and one of the cured patients had a prosthetic valve. These four patients were excluded from the analysis of native valve vegetation size and outcome (see Table 15.1).

Table 15.1 Mortality as a function of valvular vegetation size in a study on right-sided endocarditis (*Source:* Hecht and Berger[4])

Vegetation size (cm)	Number of episodes	Mortality (%)
≤ 1	19	0
1.1–2	61	2
> 2	18	33

Evidently the risk of dying increases with increasing size of the vegetation, and the difference in risk between the last group and the first two combined is highly significant.

The authors also analysed whether prolonged fever, lasting more than 3 weeks, had any adverse effect on outcome, but they did not find any such association.

This study is also instructive because it highlights the difficulties in performing epidemiological studies in the clinic, even under optimum circumstances. Of the original intended 132 episodes to be analysed, 34 episodes had to be excluded for different reasons – a dropout rate that I would describe as quite normal. One could speculate how the 30 episodes in which the patient left the hospital too early would have influenced the result. The article does not indicate how long they stayed in the hospital, but the median number of treatment days for those who died was around 10. It might be assumed that those who left had less severe disease, and that their inclusion would decrease the overall CFR, but in the absence of any data on those patients this must remain speculation.

A study from Kenya[5] attempted to assess whether any simple clinical signs or symptoms could predict the outcome in children coming to hospital with malaria. It looked at all 1866 children admitted with a primary diagnosis of *Plasmodium falciparum* malaria in the period 1989 to 1991. Of these, 18 children arrived in a moribund state, and four died from other causes. After these had been excluded from the study, 1844 children remained, 64 of whom died, with a CFR of 3.5% (95% CI: 2.7–4.3). The upper age limit for inclusion as a child was not stated in the article.

A number of conditions observable at admission were recorded, including coma, anaemia, convulsions, haemoglobinuria, jaundice, etc. Since this is a cohort study, one can calculate the risk of dying in patients who had, and who did not have, every specific condition. The ones that were found to be statistically significant in a univariate χ^2 analysis are listed in Table 15.2.

Table 15.2 Signs, symptoms and laboratory findings at admittance related to risk of dying from *Plasmodium falciparum* malaria in Kenyan children (*Source*: Marsh et al.[5])

Criterion	Number of patients with data available	Prevalence	Deaths	RR (95% CI)
Coma	1844	185	31	12.6 (7.2–22)
Respiratory distress	1833	251	35	9.4 (5.5–16.2)
Hypoglycaemia	698	92	20	5.4 (2.9–10.2)
Circulatory collapse	1844	7	5	47.7 (7.8–293.5)
Repeated convulsions	1842	338	23	2.9 (1.7–4.9)
Jaundice	1806	84	10	4.6 (2.2–9.4)

One can see that shock was very uncommon, and also that blood glucose was only measured in about half of the patients.

The authors then proceeded with a multivariate analysis of their findings, but they ran into a problem which is not uncommon. Data on different criteria were missing for a number of patients, and they were not missing for the same patients. This is one of the problems of a detailed multivariate analysis, since ideally the majority of subjects should have values for all of the variables examined. If one large group of patients has missing values for one variable, and another large group has missing values for another, then the power of a multivariate analysis will be very weak. In this study, the investigators did not have a working blood gas and pH meter during part of the study, and they were unable to measure blood glucose levels in most patients. In the final analysis, they therefore excluded blood glucose as a risk factor.

The logistic regression analysis yielded three independent risk factors for dying from falciparum malaria, namely impaired consciousness, respiratory distress and jaundice. The authors concluded that children who have impaired consciousness or respiratory distress, or both, represent 84% of the fatal cases, and that these are the ones in most urgent need of attention and treatment.

DOSE AND SEVERITY OF DISEASE

An important issue in the discussion of natural history of infectious diseases is whether a higher dose at infection leads to a more severe disease. Since most pathogens divide and multiply at a high rate, it is not self-evident that the actual number received is of any significance – the number will increase rapidly anyway. In the example in Chapter 14 involving volunteers ingesting

Salmonella typhii, there did not seem to be any such correlation, even if the average incubation period was shorter with higher doses.

The relationship between dose, measured as the degree of contact between case and susceptible individual, and severity of measles infection was studied in an area of Senegal.[6] The foundation for the study was a surveillance system operating in 30 villages with a total population of around 24 000. The villages were made up of compounds, where on average 14 people lived, although some could have over 100 inhabitants. Within each compound there were a number of households (with eight members on average), defined as a group of people who normally ate together, and each household in turn occupied a number of huts (2.5 individuals per hut on average). Measles cases in children were reported by their parents, and clinically confirmed by a physician. No serological samples were taken. Cases that were not seen by a physician were still included if they were linked epidemiologically to other known cases in the same compound or the same village.

The investigators wanted to study the case fatality rate for measles in this population. One then has to decide how late after the disease death could occur and still be regarded as being due to the infection. In studies on measles, deaths up to 6 weeks after the appearance of rash are usually attributed to the infection, and this limit was chosen here, too.

Between 1983 and 1986, 1500 cases of measles were reported, and 98 of these cases died within 6 weeks, for an overall CFR of 6.5%. The CFR varied quite widely with age, from over 10% for children aged between 6 months and 3 years to 0% for children over 10 years of age and adults. Simply dividing the cases into those younger or older than 41 months (3.5 years) at onset gives us the CFR values shown in Table 15.3.

The first case diagnosed in a compound was regarded as primary, and cases that appeared in the same compound 6–16 days after the primary case were described as secondary. Of course there is always some uncertainty about the actual source of the secondary cases, as they could also have become infected outside the compound, but if the onset of disease fell within the right serial interval, they were still included in the study. If there were several simultaneous primary cases in a compound, the source of exposure for each secondary case was assumed to be the closest one (i.e. in the same hut, same household, or same compound, in that order). One can appreciate how

Table 15.3 Case fatality rate (CFR) in measles by age in an area of Senegal (*Source*: Garenne and Aaby[6])

Age (months)	Cases	Deaths	CFR (%)
4–41	735	87	12
⩾ 42	765	11	1.4

meticulously data for time of onset and location of each case must be collected in a study such as this.

For 190 cases there was no adequate information on exposure. Of the remaining cases, 402 were classified as primary and 908 as secondary. For each of the secondary cases the type of exposure to its primary case was assessed. The CFRs according to type of exposure are listed in Table 15.4.

Table 15.4 The same study as in Table 15.3, now showing case fatality rate (CFR) in secondary cases depending on place of exposure

Exposure	Cases	Deaths	CFR (%)
Secondary in:			
Compound	203	11	5.4
Household	310	22	7.1
Hut	395	39	9.9

If we set the risk of dying to be equal to 1 if a child was exposed in the compound only, then the relative risks for the secondary cases become 7.1/5.4 = 1.31 for exposure in a household, and 9.9/5.4 = 1.83 for exposure in a hut. These differences are significant, and point to the fact that closeness of contact affects the severity of the disease, measured as fatality.

However, let us use this study for a recapitulation of confounders and how to control for them. Table 15.3 showed that age was strongly inversely associated with risk of dying. If we divide the secondary cases according to how they were exposed, it seems likely, for example, that infants would be more likely to be exposed in a hut than while running around in the compound. We thus have every reason to believe that place of exposure would also be associated with age, and that age of the secondary case could be a confounder.

We can therefore retabulate the secondary cases, this time drawing up two tables, one for children aged 41 months or less (see Table 15.5) and one for those aged 42 months or more (see Table 15.6).

The effect of exposure thus seems even more pronounced in the older children. (One should observe, however, that only one case that was infected in

Table 15.5 Case fatality rate (CFR) in secondary cases aged 4 to 41 months (RR = relative risk)

Exposure	Cases	Deaths	CFR (%)	RR (compound = 1)
Secondary in:				
Compound	91	10	11.0	1.0
Household	158	18	11.4	1.04
Hut	189	33	17.5	1.59

Table 15.6 Case fatality rate (CFR) in secondary cases aged 42 months or over (RR = relative risk)

Exposure	Cases	Deaths	CFR (%)	RR (compound = 1)
Secondary in:				
Compound	112	1	0.9	1.00
Household	152	4	2.6	2.89
Hut	206	6	2.9	3.22

the compound died in the older group, and that the calculation of RRs is quite uncertain; the confidence intervals would be wide.)

If we want to avoid having two tables, and just give one age-adjusted RR for each type of contact, we can use the Mantel–Haenszel (MH) method described in Chapter 9. The cases exposed in the compound would form the baseline group, and we would have two age groups for exposure in the household and two for exposure in huts. For the two groups exposed in the household, the MH weight for the younger children would be as follows:

$$w_{4-41} = 10 \times \frac{158}{91 + 158} = 6.34$$

which is read as 'for the children in the younger group, the weight is calculated as the number of deaths in the baseline group (10) multiplied by all cases in the household group (158) divided by the sum of cases in the two groups (91 + 158)'.

For children in the older group, the weight becomes:

$$w_{42-} = 1 \times \frac{152}{112 + 152} = 0.58$$

We can see that the weight for the RR in the older group is much lower, due to the fact that there was only one case in the baseline (i.e. compound) group.

Each weight is multiplied by its corresponding RR, and the overall RR for dying after exposure in the household compared with the risk of dying after exposure in the compound, regardless of age, becomes:

$$RR_{MH} = \frac{1.04 \times 6.34 + 2.89 \times 0.58}{6.34 + 0.58} = 1.20$$

Thus it is clearly lower than the crude RR given by Table 15.4, which was 1.31. In a similar manner, the RR_{MH} for dying after exposure in the hut is calculated to be 1.73, which is also lower than the crude relative risk of 1.83. In this example, exposure was thus confounded by age, in that the children who had the closest exposure also tended to be the younger children.

This study shows a clear relationship between dose and severity. It was performed as a cohort study, in which all cases of measles were followed up. An alternative approach would have been to perform a case–control study, where the children who died would have been the cases, and a sample of the surviving cases could be taken as controls (the terminology gets rather muddled in a situation like this). The pattern of exposure could then have been compared in the two groups.

OTHER COFACTORS FOR SEVERITY

The list of cofactors that influence the course of an infection once it has been established is very long. This book looks at only a few of these, first because they are usually studied using research methods that have already been described here and which are not unique to infectious disease epidemiology, and secondly, because they really belong more in a textbook of infectious disease medicine. Panum's study and the study from Senegal address age, but factors such as nutritional status, immune competence, sex, ethnicity, access to treatment, concurrent chronic diseases, etc., also play major roles.

SUMMARY

The natural history of an infectious disease is usually studied in cohorts of patients who are followed over time. There is a potential risk of bias if only hospitalized patients are selected, since asymptomatic or mild cases will go undetected.

The study of incubation periods for diseases that are spread from person to person requires careful mapping of the chain of transmission in the population.

Prognostic factors for the outcome of an infection are usually studied in cohorts as well, where clinical and laboratory findings early in the course of disease are compared with different outcomes.

The previous chapter showed that attack rate is associated with dose. There is also an indication that a higher dose may lead to more severe disease.

A large number of cofactors will influence the course of an infection once it has become established in a patient.

REFERENCES

1. Panum PL. Observations made during the epidemic of measles on the Faroe Islands in the year 1846. Reprinted in Buck Q, Llopis A, Nájera E, Terris M, (eds): *The challenge of epidemiology*. Washington, DC: Pan American Health Organization, Scientific Publication No. 505, 1989: 37–41.
2. Salas R, de Manzione N, Tesh RB *et al.* Venezuelan haemorrhagic fever. *Lancet* 1991; **338:** 1033–6.
3. McCarthy N, Giesecke J. Incidence of Guillain–Barré syndrome following infection with *Campylobacter jejuni. Am J Epidemiol* 2001; **153:** 610–14.

4. Hecht SR, Berger M. Right-sided endocarditis in injecting drug users. Prognostic factors in 102 episodes. *Ann Intern Med* 1992; **117**: 560–66.

5. Marsh K, Forster D, Waruiru C *et al.* Indicators of life-threatening malaria in African children. *N Engl J Med* 1995; **332**: 1399–404.

6. Garenne M, Aaby P. Pattern of exposure and measles mortality in Senegal. *J Infect Dis* 1990; **161**: 1088–94.

Chapter 16
Seroepidemiology

Here we deal with serological tools for epidemiology, starting with a very brief description of the immune response and of laboratory methods. Titres and cut-off values are discussed, and some examples of seroepidemiological studies are given. Some potential biases are mentioned, in particular the age cohort effect.

For most diseases, markers exist that can be measured in the laboratory, (e.g. for diabetes, thyrotoxicosis, myocardial infarction, renal failure, etc.). Laboratory markers are of course also important in the diagnosis of many infectious diseases, such as the pattern of liver enzymes in hepatitis or the infected red blood cells in malaria. However, the use of serological markers of infection adds another dimension to laboratory diagnosis. They may tell us not only about the disease that the patient has at present, but also about diseases that he has had in the past, in many instances decades ago, and from which he is now fully recovered. This provides us with an important tool for epidemiological studies.

When the body encounters a bacterium or a virus for the first time, a very complex immunological reaction is triggered to combat and control the spread of the pathogen. The details of this mechanism are being revealed in laboratories around the world at an amazing pace, and I shall not go into any detailed discussion here – that topic already fills many books much more voluminous than this one. Instead, I shall merely give a brief outline. Any substance that the immune system of the body recognizes as being foreign is called an *antigen* (i.e. something that generates an anti-reaction). It could be a protein, a polysaccharide, a lipid, or some combination of these. Usually one does not call an entire bacterium an antigen, but rather each of its sub-components. The immune system reacts to an antigen in two main ways. One is called *cellular immunity*, and consists of the production of specific white blood cells that are capable of recognizing and destroying the particular antigen. The other works by the production of another type of white blood cell, called a B-lymphocyte, which produce specific proteins called *antibodies* that bind to the antigen. This reaction is termed the 'humoral immune response'. The binding may incapacitate the antigen, but it also makes it easier for other white blood cells to destroy it.

The first type of immune response is of relatively little diagnostic and epidemiological use. Cellular immunity has hitherto been difficult to assay, even if current developments in this field are rapid. Its main use has been to test for exposure to tuberculosis bacteria. Infection with *Mycobacterium tuberculosis,* or with its relatives such as the BCG vaccine, gives rise to a cellular response that can be assessed by the injection of a small amount of purified antigen (from killed mycobacteria) just under the surface of the skin. Someone who has been infected with the tuberculosis bacterium or with BCG (or with a number of other mycobacteria that exist in our environment) will react to the injection by producing a small area of inflammation at the site. The size of this inflammatory reaction is believed to correlate with the degree of immunological reaction.

In contrast, the humoral immune response has widespread diagnostic and epidemiological applications. Several different classes of antibodies exist, but the two most important ones for epidemiology are called IgM and IgG ('Ig' stands for 'immunoglobulin'). This class division is concerned with the overall structure of the antibodies, but within each class there exist huge numbers of antibodies of differing *specificity* (i.e. that preferentially bind to different specific antigens). During and after an infection, the proportion of all antibodies that have a specificity for just the antigens of that pathogen will increase.

The presence and amount of antibody to an antigen can be measured in the laboratory: One small well in an array of wells on a clear plastic plate is coated with a small amount of the purified antigen from some external source. A serum sample from the patient is placed in the same well. If there are antibodies in the sample directed against the antigen, they will bind. The well is then carefully washed to get rid of everything that does not bind to the antigen coat. Note that there must be an excess of antigen in the well, or some of the antibodies which we want to measure will not find anywhere to bind, and will be washed out.

In order to visualize the amount of antibody that has bound to the coat, we need a marker of some kind. This is usually obtained by first injecting rabbits with human immunoglobulin (a mixture of many different antibodies), which their immune system will recognize as foreign, and against which they will form their own rabbit antibodies. These anti-human rabbit antibodies are then taken out of the rabbit and chemically bound to an enzyme that is able to convert some colourless substance into a coloured one.

The now enzyme-linked rabbit antibodies are placed in the original well, and they will bind to the human antibodies that were already stuck to the antigen. After another careful washing, a solution of the colourless chemical substance is placed in the well. The amount of substance that is converted by the enzyme into a coloured substance can be measured in a spectrophotometer. The photometer reading will be a measure of the amount of enzyme in the well, and thus of the amount of anti-human rabbit antibodies, and thus of the amount of the antibody that we originally wanted to measure. This is a simplified description of a procedure called enzyme-linked immunosorbent assay (ELISA or EIA), which may also be performed in other ways, and which is currently the standard method of measuring the amount of antibody against a specific antigen.

TITRES

The ELISA method can be used to obtain directly a quantitative value for the amount of antibody. Older serological methods (of which several exist, such as haemagglutination, haemagglutination inhibition, complement fixation, etc.) usually give only a 'yes' or 'no' answer to the question of whether or not there is antibody in the sample. With these methods, quantification is achieved by diluting the serum sample. One starts with a small amount of the undiluted sample (dilution 1:1). If this is positive for antibody, one takes another small volume of the sample and dilutes, most often by 1:2 or 1:10. If this new sample is again positive, one tests the next dilution step, and so on until the last diluted sample is negative in the serological test. The highest dilution which tests positive is called the titre, and this is regarded as a quantitative value of the amount of antibody in the original sample. In the example given in Table 16.1, the titre would be 1:32 (sometimes expressed as the inverse, i.e. 32).

Table 16.1 Example of results of antibody testing in a dilution series (one often checks one dilution step 'extra' to make sure that the first negative titre was not just a laboratory error)

Dilution	Test result
1 : 1	+
1 : 2	+
1 : 4	+
1 : 8	+
1 : 16	+
1 : 32	+
1 : 64	−
1 : 128	−

Note that a titre value of 1/1000 is said to be *higher* than a value of 1/10, even though 0.001 is really smaller than 0.1.

Calculation of the average titre for a group of subjects has to be done in a special manner, since a dilution series such as the one above gives a type of exponential scale, with each step being twice as large as the previous one, and one cannot simply average the values to obtain a group mean. Instead one calculates the *geometrical mean titre* or GMT. An ordinary mean is defined as the sum of all values divided by the number of subjects, but a geometrical mean is obtained by multiplying all of the values, and then taking the nth root of this number, where n is the number of subjects.

If the titres in a group of four subjects were 1/32, 1/64, 1/32 and 1/128, the geometrical mean titre would thus be as follows:

$$\text{GMT} = \sqrt[4]{\frac{1}{32} \times \frac{1}{64} \times \frac{1}{32} \times \frac{1}{128}} = \frac{1}{54}$$

Another way of performing the same calculation is to take the logarithms of each titre, add them, divide by the number of subjects, and then exponentiate the result.

Either formula can only be used when everyone has a titre. If there are seronegative samples in the series, the GMT cannot be calculated this way.

SENSITIVITY AND SPECIFICITY

One of the most important issues in serology concerns the interpretation of borderline results. We touched upon this question in Chapter 8, but I shall consider it in more detail here.

If a serological test always identified the correct antibody (high sensitivity) and never identified any other substances in the serum (high specificity), then there would be no problem. However, in reality this does not happen. Suppose we tested for antibody in a number of people who we knew had had a certain infection. The concentrations in their blood would not be exactly the same for all of them – some would have high titres and some would have low ones. The pattern is often as illustrated in Figure 16.1.

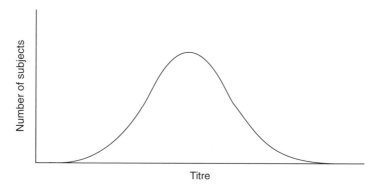

Figure 16.1 Example of distribution of antibody titres in a sample of immunized subjects.

If we performed the same test on another sample of people whom we (in some mysterious way) knew had not had the disease, we would probably obtain the curve shown in Figure 16.2.

The reason for this is that it is impossible to avoid non-specific reactions in a serological test. There will always be other proteins in serum that will

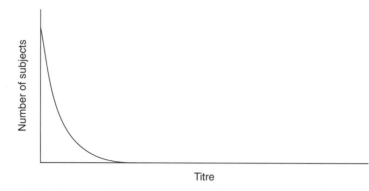

Figure 16.2 Example of distribution of non-specific titres in a sample of non-immunized subjects.

stick to the antigen coat in the ELISA to some degree. This amount of non-specific reactivity will vary between individuals.

If we now used this test in a real population, where some had antibody and some did not, we would obtain a distribution of titre values that was a superimposition of the two curves (see Figure 16.3).

How should we deal with the titre values where the two distributions overlap? If we say that everyone with a titre value above L is seropositive, then we will include a number with strong non-specific reactions (high sensitivity and lower specificity). If we instead choose H as our cut-off point, then we shall not obtain any non-specific reactions, but we will exclude some of the true seropositives (high specificity and lower sensitivity). In reality, too, the true shapes of the two curves are seldom known perfectly, and the size of the overlap zone will be uncertain.

There are no definite rules for choice of cut-off point, and it must depend on the reason for performing the test. Reports from good serological studies should always include an account of how the cut-off point was set.

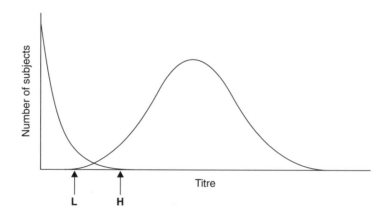
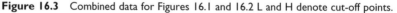

Figure 16.3 Combined data for Figures 16.1 and 16.2 L and H denote cut-off points.

TIME AND TITRES

The different classes of immunoglobulins usually appear at different times during and after an infection. IgM antibodies can be detected first, but they also disappear from the patient's serum rather rapidly after the infection. IgG antibodies appear later, but usually remain in the serum for much longer. This time pattern can sometimes be used to assess how recent an infection is. For example, IgM antibodies to hepatitis B virus are a certain diagnostic test for acute infection.

Antibodies of the IgM type can seldom be detected earlier than 1 week to 10 days after the infection. IgG antibody titres may still be quite low during the acute disease. In these instances one makes use of so-called paired sera, in which a new sample is taken about 2 weeks after the first one. If there is a clear increase in titre between these two tests, this is taken as an indication or proof that the patient has had the infection in question. In most cases a four-fold raise in titre is required, (e.g. from 1:16 in the first test to 1:64 in the second), but this rule may vary for different diseases. For some diseases, where titres in the general population are known to be low, a single high IgG titre can be used to make a diagnosis. For example, a titre against *Legionella* bacteria of more than 1:128 is often considered to indicate recent infection (at least if the patient has had symptoms suggestive of Legionnaires' disease).

USAGE

Serology has two main uses in epidemiology. The first is in cross-sectional studies of seroprevalence in different populations. Such studies may be rendered more analytical by relating seroprevalence to factors such as age, geography, lifestyle, etc., and one example is given by the herpes simplex type 1 data described in Chapter 9, where an attempt was made to relate seroprevalence to changes in sexual behaviour. Another example comes from a Turkish study that attempted to elucidate the risk factors for having become infected with hepatitis E virus.[1]

In a previous study of cardiovascular morbidity in five regions of Turkey, sera from 8000 people had been collected together with demographic data from interviews. Of these, 300 samples from each region were selected at random. Demographic data were missing for 51 samples, and for some reason only 201 samples were used from one of the regions. The samples were tested with an ELISA in which the antigen had been produced by a recombinant technique. In total, 80 of the 1350 samples tested were positive for hepatitis E antibody for an overall seroprevalence of 5.9%. Eight putative risk factors were then first analysed against seropositivity in a univariate analysis. Table 16.2 gives an example from this analysis, where the covariate studied was the number of children that each study subject had.

Using the methods described in the previous chapters, we can calculate the

Table 16.2 Seropositivity by number of children in a study on hepatitis E markers in Turkey: univariate analysis (*Source*: Thomas et al.[1])

Number of children	Number of subjects	Seropositive (%)
0	497	3.4
1–2	481	5.2
>2	372	10.2

ORs for being seropositive depending on the number of children. The table is not set up in the usual 2×2 fashion, but it can easily be converted. In the first group, the seroprevalence was 3.4%. If 497 is multiplied by 0.034, the result is 16.898, and we can thus guess that there were 17 seropositive and 480 seronegative subjects in this group. Similarly, $481 \times 0.052 = 25.012$, so there were probably 25 positive and 456 negative subjects in the group with one or two children. These figures are entered in a 2×2 table, the confidence interval is calculated according to the method for case–control studies described in Chapter 5, and the P-value can be calculated by the χ^2 method detailed in Chapter 7. The group with more than two children is then compared with the baseline group by making a new 2×2 table. The resulting ORs, 95% confidence intervals and P values are as follows:

1–2 children vs. none: OR = 1.5 (95% CI: 0.8, 3.1), $P = 0.171$;
> 2 children vs. none: OR = 3.2 (95% CI: 1.7, 6.2), $P < 0.001$.

There seems to be a strong association between 'having three or more children' and being seropositive.

The factors that were found to be significantly associated with seropositivity at the 5% level in the univariate analysis were higher age, lower educational level, higher number of children, having antibody to hepatitis C, and place of residence. The authors then performed a logistic regression analysis, in which confounding would be controlled for, and found that the number of children disappeared as a significant risk factor. With all probability, this was due to confounding by age, as younger people generally have fewer children than older ones. The most interesting finding in this study was that no subject under the age of 20 years was seropositive, whereas for hepatitis A, which is also an enteric infection, the great majority of people in Turkey will have antibody by the age of 20 years.

Another example comes from a study of hepatitis B infection among expatriates in South East Asia.[2] The prevalence of markers for hepatitis B infection was related to length of stay in South-East Asia for 133 men. The results are shown in Table 16.3.

The risk of having become infected obviously increased with length of stay, and the incidence seems to have been about 10% per year of stay, but no attempt was made to control for confounders in this study, and we must

Table 16.3 Prevalence of markers to hepatitis B virus (HBV) among expatriates in South-East Asia (*Source*: Dawson et al.[2])

Length of stay (years)	Proportion with HBV markers	Percentage
< 1	0/11	0
1	2/22	9
2	6/34	18
3	3/19	16
4	9/19	47
≥ 5	12/28	43

assume that the men were similar in all respects apart from length of stay. The authors suggested that heterosexual intercourse was the most probable source of infection. Only one in five of the infected individuals had a history of jaundice, so if the study had been based on diagnosed cases only, the estimate of risk for infection would have been very different.

The second use of seroepidemiology is to follow the incidence of an infection, either in a defined cohort or by means of repeated samples from a larger population. In the latter case, the incidence is estimated from changes in prevalence between the samples. An advantage of seroepidemiology in this situation is that it obviates the need for continuous surveillance of cases – the cumulative incidence between two time points will be directly evident from the serological data. In addition, subclinical cases will be included.

A somewhat different example of this method is given by the US study of a measles outbreak just after the blood donation drive already cited in Chapter 14.[3] During the months after a blood collection drive had taken place in a university in New England, a measles epidemic occurred in a couple of dormitories. A total of 90 students who had donated blood volunteered to take part in the study, of whom eight were clinically diagnosed cases of measles. You will remember from Chapter 14 that there was a strong association between pre-exposure antibody levels and risk of clinical disease. However, in this study the authors were also able to demonstrate a booster effect in already vaccinated students who did not develop clinical measles. A total of 18 non-case students who had donated blood agreed to have their blood tested after the outbreak. The laboratory method used was a 'plaque reduction test', which measures the extent to which the patient's serum is able to inhibit measles virus infection of a cell culture. Eleven of the 18 students who had antibody titres below 1000 in their blood donation samples showed a fourfold or higher boost in titre after the outbreak, whereas none of the seven students with titres above 1000 pre-exposure showed a fourfold rise. This study is one of several that clearly demonstrate the existence of a natural booster effect, with a rise in antibody titres after exposure in people who are already immune to a disease.

The importance of natural boosters in maintaining immunity over long periods is controversial. This issue is receiving increased attention with the introduction of vaccine programmes that aim to eliminate or eradicate diseases. Whereas until now immunized individuals have still been exposed to wild viruses or bacteria circulating in society and have thus had an opportunity to receive natural boosters, this re-exposure will disappear after a successful elimination programme, and the concern is whether the vaccine-induced immunity will still be lifelong. It may well be that a vaccine dose in adulthood will be necessary to maintain a country free from many of the diseases that are covered by a general child vaccination programme.

Seroepidemiology is also used extensively in the evaluation of vaccine effects, as we shall see in Chapter 19.

BIAS

Inevitably, many seroepidemiological studies are being performed on available material (i.e. most often frozen serum samples). There is always a risk of bias when using this method. Who are the patients whose blood is saved in a serum bank? What was the reason for the test in the first place?

If one wants to make estimates of seropositivity in the general population, one should remember that samples of sera in a serum bank were nearly always taken for clinical reasons. Patients who have a blood test taken differ from the general population in that they are usually ill in some way. The probability of visiting a physician varies greatly with age and sex, and in most developed countries a serum bank of random samples will be skewed towards older ages. Young women may have blood taken in connection with pregnancy, but men between 20 and 50 years of age may not see a doctor for decades. Stored sera from children will often show a disproportionately high number of very young and much older children, and the age groups at which children can defend themselves but still not understand the necessity of the test will be under-represented.

It is also doubtful to what extent sera from healthy blood donors can be used to make population estimates. In countries where blood donation is unpaid, blood donors will tend to be concerned and responsible individuals, and thus probably healthier than average, whereas the reverse may be true in countries with paid donors. Few sociological studies have been conducted to characterize blood donors.

Researchers approaching epidemiology from the laboratory perspective have a tendency to regard their blood samples, bacterial clones or viral strains as 'populations', (e.g. when talking about the prevalence of some marker in their collection of bacteria). In the strict sense, 100 bacterial cultures of course constitute some type of population, but this use of the word deflects thinking and may mislead the unwary.

THE AGE COHORT EFFECT

This is a rather special type of fallacy which quite often arises in seroepide-miological studies. If we test a random sample of the population for, say, anti-body to *Helicobacter pylori*, and we find that seroprevalence increases with age, what does that tell us about the present incidence in various age groups?

If a cohort of subjects are followed over time with repeated serologies, it will be easy to calculate the yearly incidence of infection. However, matters become more complicated if we instead choose to perform a cross-sectional study right now, by measuring the percentage of seropositive individuals in different age groups. For many diseases, such as hepatitis A or herpes simplex type 1, such a study will show an increase in the proportion with markers (i.e. seroprevalence) with increasing age. If those who are now 10 years old have a seroprevalence of 10% and those who are now 30 years old have one of 35%, does this mean that 25% of today's 10-year-olds will contract the disease in the next 20 years? The answer is, not necessarily. If overall expo-sure to the pathogen is decreasing over time, perhaps as a consequence of improved hygiene, this means that those who have lived longer were more exposed when they were young. As an example, let us consider an imaginary disease which is becoming rarer with time. Let us assume that up until 50 years ago the risk of catching this disease was 5% per year, if one was sus-ceptible. Since then, the risk has decreased by 0.1% per year, so that it has been 0.1% during the last year. The current seroprevalence by age in the pop-ulation would then be as shown in Figure 16.4.

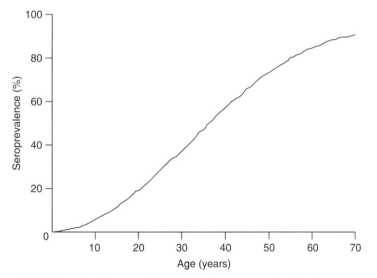

Figure 16.4   Example of seroprevalence vs. age in a cross-sectional study.

From this figure, it seems that the maximum age-specific incidence of this disease is for ages between 30 and 40 years, and that almost everyone will have had the disease by the time they reach the age of 70. In reality, the shape of the curve is due to the decreasing risk with time. What it in fact shows is that the older subjects were much more exposed when they were young. If the present incidence of 0.1% per year remained constant for the next 70 years, the curve for a true cohort study of today's newborn would show an almost linear increase with age, and a cumulative incidence at the age of 70 years of just under 7%.

This fallacy is known as the *age cohort effect*, and it is something to look out for whenever one uses a cross-section of data from different age groups to make predictions about what will happen when the present-day population progresses through these age groups. For many Western countries, the age curve for seroprevalence against hepatitis A looks something like the above graph, even though the incidence of hepatitis A is now quite low. Since there was more transmission of the infection several decades ago, the graph will display a sort of 'seroepidemiological archaeology'.

In the study from Turkey cited earlier, the authors point out that the peculiar age distribution of antibody to hepatitis E virus could be a cohort effect if transmission of this agent decreased sharply about 20 years ago.

SUMMARY

Serology provides an important tool for infectious disease epidemiology, making it possible to measure the incidence and cumulative incidence of infections in different populations.

Antibody levels are often expressed as titres, and these require special mathematics when groups are to be compared.

All serological tests suffer to a greater or lesser extent from problems with non-specific reactions. By shifting the value for the cut-off point, one can increase either sensitivity or specificity (but not both).

Cross-sectional studies of seroprevalence can reveal risk factors for infection and suggest possible transmission routes, but cohort studies with frequent sampling of blood may be even more valuable in this respect, since the time for seroconversion will be better described.

Collecting blood from a random population sample is always difficult, and it may be tempting to use stored serum samples instead. In this case one should be aware of the different biases possible.

The age-cohort effect is a special problem with cross-sectional studies in which seroprevalence is related to age. Has general exposure been decreasing with time? If so, the curve of prevalence for age will not show the age-dependent risk of infection facing the present-day population.

REFERENCES

1. Thomas DL, Mahley RW, Badur S, Palaoglu KE, Quinn TC. Epidemiology of hepatitis E virus infection in Turkey. *Lancet* 1993; **341:** 1561–2.

2. Dawson DG, Spivey GH, Korelitz JJ, Schmidt RT. Hepatitis B: risk to expatriates in South-East Asia. *BMJ* 1987; **294:** 547.
3. Chen RT, Markowitz LE, Albrecht P *et al.* Measles antibody: re-evaluation of protective titers. *J Infect Dis* 1990; 162: 1036–42.

Chapter 17
The study of
contact patterns

Here the concept of contact patterns is addressed in more depth. Methods for depicting such patterns are described, and some examples are given of the research methods used to investigate how people mix.

As has been mentioned repeatedly throughout this book, the epidemiology of infectious diseases is not only about the properties of various pathogens and their hosts, but also to a great extent about contact patterns in the population. This is of course especially true for diseases that are spread from person to person either, directly or via an intermediate host. In the prevaccination era, measles epidemics in Western Europe always started several weeks after school began in the autumn, and although it is difficult to prove, it seems highly likely that the increased contact density when children were congregated again after having been dispersed during the summer vacation was an important factor in this timing. The reasons why the incidence of most upper respiratory tract infections (e.g. streptococcal angina, diphtheria and even meningococcal meningitis) is always highest during the winter months have been discussed. Some believe that the lower humidity of room air in winter makes the mucosal surfaces more vulnerable to attacks, but an equally plausible explanation is that people tend to meet at closer range indoors during the cold season (i.e. their contact pattern changes).

At a basic level, an infectious disease that is spread from person to person cannot persist unless the infectious cases meet someone susceptible before they themselves have recovered. In terms of the pathogen, this means that an infection that is spread readily in daily social contacts does not have to be very long-lasting, as an infectious case is almost certain to meet a susceptible individual within a day or two. However, for sexually transmitted infections contacts between a case and a new partner may be few and far between, and these infections therefore have to have a very long period of infectivity, often of the order of months or years.

Continuing this line of reasoning, it seems unlikely that the highly infectious and highly immunogenic (i.e. leading to a very good protective immune response) diseases such as measles or smallpox could have existed in human populations during the millenniums when we lived as hunters and gatherers. At that time, all humans lived in family or clan groups of perhaps some 100 people at the most, and with limited contact between groups.[1] If measles entered such a group it would rapidly infect almost everyone, but where would the virus go after that? The probability of a contact outside the group during the infectious period must have been low. In fact, modern data exist on measles epidemics on islands which indicate that a population of around 500 000 is necessary to maintain measles endemic.[2] The virus needs a steady influx of susceptible individuals, and in the absence of immigration this is supplied by the children who are born into the population.

For those diseases that can confer lifelong infectivity, matters are somewhat different. The viruses of the herpes group (herpes simplex, varicella, etc.) are sometimes reactivated in infected subjects as cold sores or as shingles, which are both infectious, and those infections could thus persist in much smaller populations. For examples, someone infected with chicken-pox as a child might develop shingles decades later, and subsequently infect his or her grandchildren.

Incidentally, it is just those diseases that are highly infectious and immunogenic that we call childhood diseases. In a demographically stable society, the children are the only susceptible individuals entering the population, and they will be the ones who keep the chain of infection going. There is nothing about the viruses themselves that make them especially prone to infect young children.

Another interesting consequence of changing contact patterns in society is the shift towards a higher average age at infection that has been observed for many classical childhood diseases such as polio, hepatitis A, and possibly chicken-pox. As hygiene standards improve and families get less crowded, the amount of exposure during childhood decreases, and more and more children will escape infection. This will lead to an increased proportion of cases appearing in adolescents and adults, and these will often be more severe than if the infection had been acquired in childhood.

For many infectious diseases, population density and subsequently contact density thus become important determinants of epidemiology. However, even with a given contact density there may be considerable heterogeneity in contact patterns. As was emphasized in Chapter 11, it is a highly unrealistic assumption that everyone in the population has exactly the same chance of meeting everyone else. In order to understand the epidemiology of infections better, one also needs to study contact patterns.

MATRICES AND GRAPHS

Sociologists often make use of graphs to describe the network of contacts in a group of people. They call them sociograms, and they might appear as shown in Figure 17. 1.

This graph could show which of the five people A, B, C, D and E knew

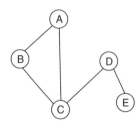

Figure 17.1 A sociogram showing the contacts between five people.

each other. In the language of graph theory, the rings (people in this case) are called *nodes,* and the lines between them are called *links.*

An alternative way of representing the same graph would be to make a *contact matrix,* as follows:

	A	B	C	D	E
A	—	I	I	0	0
B	I	—	I	0	0
C	I	I	—	I	0
D	0	0	I	—	I
E	0	0	0	I	—

A '1' shows that two people know each other, and a '0' shows that they do not. The first row, or the first column, shows that A knows B and C, but not D and E.

The above graph and matrix are both *non-directed,* which means that if A knows B, then B also knows A. If we had asked these five people who liked whom, the result might have been different (see Figure 17.2).

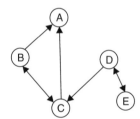

Figure 17.2 An example of a directed sociogram, in which contacts may only be unidirectional.

This graph shows that B and C both like A, as well as each other, etc., and the corresponding matrix would be as follows:

				To:		
		A	B	C	D	E
	A	—	0	0	0	0
	B	I	—	I	0	0
From:	**C**	I	I	—	0	0
	D	0	0	I	—	I
	E	0	0	0	I	—

In this case, rows and columns are not equivalent, and this matrix should be read by following a person's row from the left to see which of the others he or she likes. This graph and its corresponding matrix are both *directed*.

One problem with graphs like these is that they do not include times, and if the contact pattern is changing, one would really need a series of graphs, perhaps one for each day.

CONTACT PATTERNS AND INFECTIOUS DISEASES

It is clear that graphs and matrices such as these could be helpful for describing the spread of a disease in a population. However, there are two rather distinct possible uses.

1. The first use is the most obvious one. It is when the exact path of an infection in a population is traced from person to person, and is described in a directed graph, much as was shown in Figure 11.2, introducing the concept of R_0. In analyses of outbreaks, such graphs are often useful, not least for presenting the results to other people afterwards. Several studies on the outcome of contact tracing for STIs include graphs showing the actual chain of infection. The nodes can be given different shapes or colours to denote the person's sex, age, etc., and the links may be labelled with the time or type of contact. Furthermore, the nodes need not be individuals – they could be subgroups of people, or as in some descriptions of influenza outbreaks, entire cities. We shall call such descriptions of an actually occurring contact pattern *networks*.

2. The second use is more subtle. It attempts to describe the contact pattern in a population in the absence of any specific disease, the point being to understand what would happen if a disease with a given attack rate was introduced. How far would it spread? Which would be its most likely path? A knowledge of contact patterns would also help to clarify how endemic diseases remain in a population. Such a graph would most often depict not specific individuals, but rather some type of average contact patterns, and often at different levels (contact patterns within families, between families, in schools, at work, etc.). The links also need not be the actual contacts taking place, but rather the probability of contact over some time period.

    For a population of any size, such a graph at an individual level would be impossible to construct. Instead, one would group people according to relevant characteristics and look at the probability of contact between groups. For example, what is the probability that a 24-year-old man has sexual contact with a 21-year-old woman? What is the rate of travel from city A to city B, and what would be the risk of an influenza epidemic in A spreading to B? Graphs of this type form the basis of the stochastic models for infections described briefly in Chapter 11. We shall call descriptions of this more general type of contact pattern *contact structures*.

In mathematical terms one could say that the contact structure is the set of all possible networks that could be observed, whereas a network is the one of all these possibilities that actually did occur. Methods of studying contact patterns in real life, as well as the theoretical framework for analysing them, are still developing fields, and this is one of the most important future research areas for infectious disease epidemiology.

STUDYING NETWORKS

The basic way of assessing networks is obviously to interview people about their contacts. The contacts named are then interviewed again, and so on, in order to obtain a larger network. The size of the sample quickly becomes very large, but the approach may be possible for more restricted groups.

One such example concerning a disease that might be infectious comes from a study of the network between patients with the malignant lymphoma Hodgkin's disease in the area around Oxford in 1977.[3] It had been reported from the USA in the early 1970s that there seemed to be a high number of contacts between patients with Hodgkin's disease, which could support a role for some infectious agent with a low attack rate and a long incubation time. The relevant epidemiological question here is, of course, what is a 'high number of contacts'? Compared with what? How does one know that there had been more contacts within this group of patients than within any random group in the population? The researchers in the Oxford study tried to answer this question in a type of case–control design. A total of 97 patients who had been diagnosed with Hodgkin's disease and reported to the regional cancer registry were identified as the cases. For each case, a control was chosen to be someone who had been admitted to a hospital in the region for any reason other than cancer or chronic disease at the same time as the case patient was diagnosed. The controls were also matched to the cases with regard to sex, age, social class and geographical area.

In total, 87 of the cases, or a close relative if the case had died, could be interviewed about where they had gone to school and where they had worked. The obvious approach would then have been to ask all the controls the same questions. However, the investigators made a nice correction for possible recall bias in this study. If a case had died, they did not interview the corresponding control, but instead a close relative of the control, in order to make the collection of data as similar as possible.

A 'link' was then defined as an instance when any two people from this collection of 174 cases and controls had attended the same school or worked in the same workplace. If the findings from the American studies had been valid, there should have been more links between two Hodgkin's disease patients than between patients and controls or between two controls. From the total data set, one could calculate that the expected number of contacts between any 87 subjects should be 40.75. There were just 40 observed links between the 87 Hodgkin's disease patients, and this study therefore provided little support for any infectious aetiology.

The method of asking people about their contacts becomes considerably more sensitive when sexual contacts are the issue, which is a somewhat paradoxical situation since this is probably the one area of infectious disease epidemiology where contact patterns are most important. An example of an attempt to elucidate a network of sexual contacts by the interview method comes from a study in Iceland.[4]

In 1987 there were 35 known HIV-positive people in Iceland. Of these individuals, 22 agreed to participate in the study. They were asked to identify all of their sexual contacts during the preceding 7 years, including demographic characteristics (age, sex, place of residence, occupation, etc.), to describe the type of relationship that they had had with them, and also to indicate whether these partners knew each other and, if so, what type of relationship existed between them. The reason for the last question was mainly to be able to collate the responses from all of the subjects, making sure that the same person identified by two different subjects would not be counted as two individuals.

The 22 subjects identified a total of 91 contacts. Sixty of these contacts and 15 of the HIV-positive subjects could be connected in a network, where every node was linked to at least one other. Seven of the HIV-positive subjects could not be linked to any other infected person.

A small section of the resulting network is shown in Figure 17.3. It is easy to appreciate that the description and analysis of networks such as these are far from straightforward.

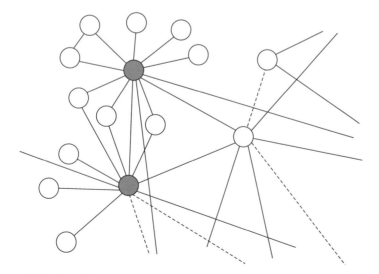

Figure 17.3 Part of a sociogram from a study on HIV-positive people in Iceland. Shaded nodes denote HIV-positive individuals, and broken lines indicate uncertainty as to whether two individuals really had sexual contact. (*Source: Haraldsdottir et al.*[4])

The study of susceptible exposure attack rates in families requires careful elucidation of the actual networks of transmission, since it is important that the tertiary and higher-order cases are differentiated from the true secondary ones. Another example is provided by Panum's measles study described in Chapter 15, where he needed to map out the exact network of the epidemic in order to calculate the incubation period.

Modern microbiology can sometimes supply tools to describe networks of infected people. This is done with some variant of 'genetic fingerprinting', by which individual strains of a bacterium or virus can be traced through a group of patients. Using restriction fragment length polymorphism (RFLP) on samples from patients in Denmark coinfected with TB and HIV, it was possible to show that during the 1990s there was only a slight overlap (2 out of 67 cases) between TB transmission in native Danes and in immigrants.[5]

STUDYING CONTACT STRUCTURES

Many important aspects of contact structures are obvious from everyday experience. For example, people are more likely to meet someone living in their neighbourhood than someone living at the other end of the country. Schools and day-care centres make good mixing places for many infections. Social class and profession influence who meets whom to a great extent. Choice of sexual partner is often restricted to roughly the same age group as one's own.

The examples in the previous section showed how actual networks between individuals could be charted. Data on contact structures could also be obtained by means of interviews, and one example is given by surveys on sexual habits in random samples of a population.

In one such survey in Sweden,[6] a random sample of young adults were asked about their age at first sexual intercourse, and also about the age of their partner. The median age of the partners for each year of first intercourse was calculated for males and for females, and the results are shown in Figure 17.4.

In Figure 17.4a, almost all of the points fall on the line for equal age, showing that the men tended to have their first intercourse with someone who was their own age (in the median). Figure 17.4b shows that the female subjects of the survey had had their first intercourse with a man who was about 2 years older than themselves. This simple survey thus revealed interesting differences in the two sexes' contact patterns at the beginning of sexual activity. One conclusion was that it must be unusual for young Swedes both to be virgins at their first intercourse, a finding which should play a role in the epidemiology of sexually transmitted diseases in these young age groups.

An interesting finding that emerges in virtually all surveys of sexual habits is that the average reported number of lifetime heterosexual partners is always higher for men than for women. Since heterosexual intercourse involves one man and one woman, the total number of female partners

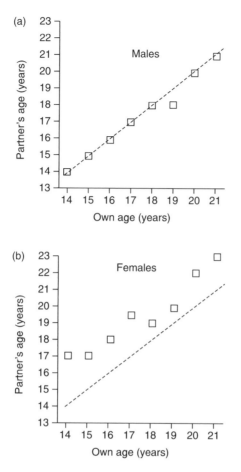

Figure 17.4 Results obtained from a Swedish study showing age at first intercourse vs. that partner's age for (a) male and (b) female respondents. Broken lines indicate where the points should have been if both partners had been of equal age. (Reproduced from Giesecke *et al.*[6] with kind permission of the publisher.)

reported by men should be the same as the total number of male partners reported by women. If there are equal numbers of the two sexes in the population, the average numbers should also be the same. This discrepancy has never been satisfactorily explained, even if a sex-related propensity to over- or under-report the number of partners could be one reason. Another explanation that has been suggested is that surveys tend to miss female sex-workers, who will have a very high number of partners, and who would raise the female average considerably if they were included.

CONTACT INTENSITY

Rate of partner change

A central concept in the epidemiological literature on sexually transmitted diseases is *rate of partner change*, or perhaps more appropriately *rate of part-*

ner acquisition. This is defined as the average number of new partners that a person will have in a given time period, most often a year. It is thus exactly the same as κ, the contact rate, in the formula for R_0 in Chapter 11.

However, there are some problems with this concept as it is being used in research on the spread of sexually transmitted diseases. The principal one is whether this characteristic exists at all. Do all people have a rate of partner change which could be given a value just like their age or height? The second problem is that even if we could assign a value for rate of partner change to a person, would this show any constancy over time? In the models discussed in Chapter 11, we just assumed an average contact rate for the population, or for large subpopulations, and this assumption could be valid even if individuals within that population changed their contact rate over time.

A person's rate of partner change is generally assessed in interviews, in which people are asked how many partners they have had in the last year, last 2 years, last 5 years, etc. From such figures one can obtain an estimate of the rate of acquisition of new partners. However, this is not straightforward, since one must take into account the fact that partnerships could extend across the boundaries of the time periods studied. For example, if a person reports that he has had two partners in the last year, this could mean that he has had two new partners, but it could equally well mean that one relationship ended and another commenced during the last year. If the previous relationship lasted for 10 years, and the new one will also last for 10 years, this person's rate of partner change will be 1/10 instead of 2. To obtain a slightly more reliable estimate, one usually subtracts the figure for partners in the last year from the figure for partners in last 5 years, and divides this by 4.

Regardless of the exact method of calculation, the problem with regard to time constancy of the value remains. There is really no way of knowing that this figure will apply to the future behaviour of this person. For example, a subject reporting a high rate of partner change could enter into a stable monogamous relationship tomorrow.

The next problem is that the figure itself is a poor descriptor of the actual contact pattern. For example, a person X who reports having two partners during the last year could have first had partner A and then partner B. If A was infected with an STI, this might be passed on to B via X. However, a not uncommon situation would be that X had a continuing relationship with A during the year, and a short contact with B. He might even have ongoing sexual relationships with them both during the year. In the latter two cases, an STI might be as likely to be passed from B via X to A as the other way around. Matters could get even more problematic if the question in the interview was 'How many new partners did you have last year?'. A person who has had several ongoing relationships, but only with 'old' partners, would answer 'zero' to this question. If his partners also had other partners, there would be a contact structure with high potential for spread of an STI in this group, even if almost all of its members reported having had no new partners during the year, and were thus assigned a rate of partner change of 0.

The epidemiologically more interesting question in the questionnaire would probably be 'How many times during the last year (or last 2, or last 5 years) did you have sexual intercourse with someone who was not your partner in the previous intercourse?'

Intensity of social contacts

An interesting discussion of the number of social contacts per day, and how this relates to transmission routes, comes from a report of a measles outbreak in a high-school in the USA.[7] On Friday 12 April 1985, a 16-year-old high-school girl developed mild cough, running nose, conjunctivitis and sore throat while still at school. Over the weekend she developed a hacking cough, but she went back to school on the Monday. The rash appeared the same day. For the next 9 days she stayed at home.

A total of 69 secondary cases in the school had onset of measles between 24 April and 3 May, with an epidemic curve just like a point-source outbreak. There were no other co-primary cases, and no third-generation cases, so the only explanation is that they were all infected by the one primary case.

A total of 58 of the secondary cases were interviewed about contacts with the girl on 12 or 15 April, and 11 of these individuals had been in the same class, studying in the cafeteria, or taking the school bus together with her. The only two places where the remaining 47 cases who were interviewed could have met her were in the cafeteria and the hallway.

For measles, the standard assumption is that a susceptible individual has to be within about 2 metres of a case to be exposed. The researchers counted how many students would pass within 2 metres of a certain point in the hallway during a break period, and found this to be 179 on average. The average number of pupils in the school on any given day was 1722. Assuming random mixing in the hallway, the probability of any student passing the primary case during a 5-minute break would be $179/1722 = 0.1$. There were 10 breaks during the day, so the probability of contact at any of these breaks would be $1 - (1-0.1)^{10} = 0.65$ (remember the method of calculating risk of transmission for gonorrhoea discussed in Chapter 14). We could therefore guess that 65% of the secondary cases, or 45 pupils, could have had contact with the primary case on 15 April, when she was probably at the peak of her infectivity.

However, the probability that they would all have had contact with her is vanishingly small, at 0.65^{69}, or 1.2×10^{-13}.

The main point about this study is that by analysing the contact pattern, it shows that the assumption that 2 metres is the effective zone of contact must be wrong. The measles virus must have spread further through the air in the school.

TYPE OF MIXING

Even if the concept of rate of partner change is quite problematic, it is still frequently used in STI epidemiology. This is due to the fact that different contact structures according to rate of partner change give rise to very different epidemic situations.

In the first instance, consider a situation where people with a certain rate of partner change mostly or only have contacts with people with the same rate. Those who have a high rate would have contact with others with high rate, and those with a low rate would have contact with others with a low rate. This pattern is called preferential or assortative mixing. If an STI entered this population, it would quickly spread among the high-rate individuals, but it might well be that the contact rate among large groups of the population would be too low to sustain even an endemic level of the disease (using the terminology of Chapter 11, R_0 would be below 1 in these groups). Cases of the disease in low-rate individuals would then mostly occur in those rare instances when a high-rate and a low-rate person had contact with each other. The disease would only remain endemic within the group of people with high rates, and if this group was small compared with the total population, the overall endemic prevalence could be low. A group of people who have a high enough rate of partner change to maintain an endemic of an STI is often called a *core group* in the STI literature.

A second type of contact structure would be one in which the rate of partner change did not influence choice of sexual partner at all. This is called random mixing. With such a contact structure, the initial spread of an STI would be much slower, since many of the infected individuals would be low-rate subjects and would probably not pass on the disease. However, the final endemic prevalence of the disease could be higher than in the preferential mixing scenario, since it could spread to much larger sections of the population.

Theoretically, there could also exist a type of contact structure with people actively seeking their partners from groups with a different rate of partner change to themselves. This is called dissortative mixing. From a sociological point of view, this seems like improbable behaviour. Most of the human activities that aim to create contacts between people, such as bars, dance places, clubs, etc., try to bring kindred souls together. It is difficult to imagine a social arrangement aimed at bringing together people who are as dissimilar as possible.

The contact structure according to rate of partner change is very difficult to study in conventional surveys. Although data may be readily collected on the number of partners that the subjects themselves have had, we cannot usually reach these partners with the same question. However, the strategy of contact tracing for STIs offers the possibility of obtaining such data. In a study in Gothenburg in Sweden, 400 women with chlamydia infection were asked about the number of male partners they had had in the last 6 months.[8] The distribution among these 400 women was as follows:

1 partner	2 partners	3 partners	4 or more partners
228	135	32	5

From these 400 women, it was possible to contact 400 male partners (for some of the women, no partner was found, and for some there was more than one). These men were asked the same question, and their distribution by number of partners during the last 6 months was as follows:

1 partner	2 partners	3 partners	4 or more partners
261	25	30	84

Let us pause here for just a moment to consider what these two samples represent. Is there any bias involved in choosing these 400 men and 400 women? The women were sampled out of a population of family planning and STI clinic attenders, and can be assumed to be representative of chlamydia-infected women in that population. However, the men were sampled because they were reported as contacts. A man who has had contact with many women must have a higher probability of being named as a contact than one who has only had intercourse with one woman. Thus the distribution of the 400 men in the study on reported number of partners above will be skewed to include 'too many' men who have had a high number of partners. This is quite evident from the much higher figure for men than for women reporting four partners or more.

This means that a contact matrix for these 800 people can only be interpreted for the women – that is, the matrix below should only be read along the rows from the left:

		Men				
		Number of partners in last 6 months				
		1	**2**	**3**	**≥ 4**	
Women	1	180	5	9	34	228
Number of	2	69	16	14	36	135
partners in	3	9	3	7	13	32
last 6 months	≥ 4	3	1	0	1	5
		261	25	30	84	400

Thus there were, for example, 135 women who reported having two partners in the last 6 months. Among the partners of women in that group, 69 men had only had that woman as a partner, 16 had had one more partner, 14 had had two more partners, and so on.

If women showed exclusive preferential mixing, all of the figures in the above matrix should have been on the diagonal from upper left to lower right, since a woman would only choose a partner with her own rate of partner change. On the other hand, if mixing had been completely random, the distribution along each of the four rows should have been similar, and equal to the total distribution in the row at the bottom, since all of the women should choose among the men in the same fashion, regardless of their own rate of partner change.

This is a good place to recapitulate the ideas behind the χ^2 test introduced in Chapter 7. For each of the cells in the above matrix we could calculate an expected value if the women's choice of sexual partner had been at random. In the top row, we can see that a total of 228 women reported having one partner. If the choice of partner had been random, these 228 relationships should be divided on the four columns just like the bottom row. There should thus be:

$$228 \times \frac{261}{400} = 149 \text{ women in the top left-hand corner,}$$

$$228 \times \frac{25}{400} = 14 \text{ women in the second cell of the first row,}$$

$$228 \times \frac{30}{400} = 17 \text{ women in the third cell, and}$$

$$228 \times \frac{84}{400} = 48 \text{ in the top right-hand cell.}$$

If we perform this calculation of the *expected* number (assuming random choice of partner) in each cell of the table, and then subtract these values from the corresponding value of the actual table, the result is as shown in the matrix below:

Difference between observed and expected number in each cell:

		Men			
		1	2	3	≥ 4
	1	31	−9	−8	−14
Women	2	−19	8	4	8
	3	−12	1	5	6
	≥ 4	0	1	0	0

With some imagination, one could see a tendency for the high positive values to concentrate on the diagonal and for the low or negative values to wind up off the diagonal, implying that women more often choose a man with an approximately equal rate of partner change than would be expected just by random choice. The fact that the distribution of the observed table is unlikely to be random can be demonstrated by calculating the actual χ^2 value, which gives a *P*-value of < 0.01.

RANDOM SAMPLING OF NETWORKS

Since the actual network of contacts in a population of any size is almost impossible to describe, one would need some method for obtaining a representative sample of networks from which a better understanding of the contact pattern could be gained. One such interesting strategy makes use of a type of random walk in a network, and the method has been used to study the population of Canberra, Australia.[9]

One starts with a list of all of the people in the population. From this list a number of individuals are chosen at random, and all of these subjects are interviewed and asked to list all of their contacts. From each primary person's list, one contact is chosen at random, and this secondary person is also approached and interviewed about all his or her contacts. The process could go on for an arbitrary number of steps. If resources are only available for a certain number of interviews, one has to decide whether to choose a larger group of primary subjects and restrict the interviews to secondary contacts, or to choose a smaller group initially and continue to tertiary or higher-order contacts. The first choice gives better precision in describing the average network around a person seen only from the individual's perspective, whereas the second choice increases the power to detect more complicated networks in the population – networks of which no single person may be aware.

In the Canberra study it was decided to select 60 individuals out of a total of around 200 000 as primary subjects, and to go on to tertiary contacts. Thus a total of 180 people were interviewed. They reported on average 30 links with other people in Canberra, and by asking about age, sex, occupation, etc., it became possible to describe the person-centred networks in some detail. Of all reported links, 8% were to relatives, 25% were to current or former neighbours, and 24% were to work associates. It is interesting that as many as 67% of all links were directed (i.e. A reported B as a contact, but B did not mention A).

Obviously there will be a number of people who are listed by more than one subject of the study. These were generally not interviewed, but by combining the lists of all of the interviewees it was possible to link around 6000 people in Canberra in a large network where everyone was connected to at least one other person, and where the maximum distance between any two people was six links. The core of this network obviously included the individuals interviewed (since only they had listed all of their contacts), but also 274 other individuals named by two or more study subjects, and one could speculate that the characteristics of these should be of great interest for the understanding of infection spread in a population such as this one.

SUMMARY

Contact patterns play an important role in determining the shape of epidemics and endemics. At the most basic level, frequency of contact decides which diseases could persist in a population.

Even with a given average contact rate, there may be large variations between subgroups. Simple epidemic models usually assume random mixing in the population, but this is unrealistic for most diseases.

Contact patterns can be described with methods borrowed from sociology, such as graphs and contact matrices. A network describes the actual pattern of contacts between a group of individuals, whilst a contact structure tries to describe the probability of contact between groups of individuals with certain characteristics.

The basic research method for investigating contact patterns is the interview or survey. However, subtyping of bacteria or viruses may sometimes make it possible to reconstruct the exact network through which an infection has spread.

The rate of partner change is an important concept in theoretical STI epidemiology, but its validity is unclear. Different types of mixing with regard to rate of partner change will have implications for the rate of spread and final endemic level of an infection.

REFERENCES

1. McKeown T. *The origins of human disease.* Oxford: Blackwell Scientific Publications, 1988.
2. Black FL. Measles endemicity in insular populations: critical community size and its evolutionary implication. *J Theor Biol* 1966; **11:** 207–11.
3. Smith PG, Kinlen LJ, Pike MC, Jones A, Harris R. Contacts between young patients with Hodgkin's disease. *Lancet* 1977; **2:** 59–62.
4. Haraldsdottir S, Gupta S, Anderson RM. Preliminary studies of sexual networks in a male homosexual community in Iceland. *J AIDS* 1992; **5:** 374–81.
5. Dragsted UB, Bauer J, Poulsen S, Askgaard D, Andersen AB, Lundgren JD. Epidemiology of tuberculosis in HIV-infected patients in Denmark. *Scand J Infect Dis* 1999; **31:** 57–61.
6. Giesecke J, Scalia-Tomba G-P, Göthberg M, Tüll P. Sexual behaviour related to the spread of STDs – a population-based survey. *Int J STD AIDS* 1992; **3:** 255–60.
7. Chen RT, Goldbaum GM, Wassilak SG, Markowitz LE, Orenstein WA. An explosive point-source measles outbreak in a highly vaccinated population. *Am J Epidemiol* 1989; **129:** 173–82.
8. Ramstedt K, Giesecke J, Forssman L, Granath F. Choice of sexual partner according to rate of partner change and social class of the partners. *Int J STD AIDS* 1991; **2:** 428–31.
9. Klovdahl AS. Sampling social networks: a simple approach to a difficult problem. Abstract from *Workshop on Generalizability Question for Snowball Sampling and Other Ascending Methodologies.* University of Groningen, 20–21 February 1992.

Chapter 18
Methods for deciding whether or not an illness is infectious

One of the most challenging tasks of infectious disease epidemiology is to try to decide whether a disease is infectious or not. This chapter looks at some methods that have been devised to investigate this problem. The most common method is to look for clusters in space and/or time, but an example of an ecological study is also given. In addition, one example is given of the converse, namely searching for a disease for a newly found microbe.

The series of experimental steps required to prove that a pathogen is the cause of a specific disease was first laid down by a German microbiologist called Löffler in 1883.[1] Thoughts along the same lines had been published by Henle in the 1840s and by Klebs in 1877. Löffler's supervisor was another well-known microbiologist called Koch, who had also advanced similar ideas, and the rules have become known to posterity as *Koch's postulates*. You can see them cited in slightly different versions, but Löffler's original wording was as follows:

The fulfilment of these postulates is necessary in order to demonstrate strictly the parasitic nature of a disease.

1. The organism must be shown to be constantly present in characteristic form and arrangement in the diseased tissue.

2. The organism which from its behaviour appears to be responsible for the disease must be isolated and grown in pure culture.

3. The pure culture must be shown to induce the disease experimentally.

Although the postulates are still being cited today, they are too dependent on bacteriological methods to be really useful. Nevertheless, it would probably be fair to say that most infectious disease clinicians and microbiologists still feel uneasy about calling a disease infectious on purely epidemiological grounds. They want to see and characterize the microbe responsible first.

SPACE-TIME CLUSTERS

The general idea behind epidemiological studies that aim to find out whether a disease is infectious is as follows. If a disease can be transmitted from one person to another, then cases should tend to cluster in space and time. We have already seen an example of such a study in the previous chapter, where links between cases of Hodgkin's disease were compared with links between controls. If that disease was infectious, it should be possible to observe clusters of patients, but no such clustering was found in that study.

A good example of a cluster analysis comes from a study of the skin disease pityriasis rosea in the UK.[2] During a 2-year period in the late 1970s all general practitioners within the catchment area of the dermatology department at North Staffordshire Hospital Centre were asked to refer all suspect cases of pityriasis rosea. In total, 126 patients had the diagnosis confirmed, and they were asked about the date of onset of the rash and their place of residence.

A list of all possible pairs of two patients was subsequently made. The first patient was paired with each of the other 125, the second patient with each of the remaining 124, and so on. For all such pairs of patients the distance between their homes and the time period between the respective onsets of disease were calculated. The number of all possible pairs between n subjects is $n(n-1)/2$, so in this case distances in space and in time had to be calculated for $126 \times 125/2 = 7875$ pairs of patients. The reasoning is then as follows. If the disease was *not* infectious, then there should be no correlation at all between distance in time and distance in space. The cases would appear at random in the population, and a plot of distance in time vs. geographical distance for each pair would look just like a shotgun swarm.

However, if the disease did have an infectious aetiology, then there would be a structure in such a plot, in that cases who lived close together would also have dates of onset quite close to one another. There might be several different chains of infection occurring simultaneously in the area, but these would be spread at random, and within each chain, cases would tend to cluster in space and time. Alternatively, if only one chain of infection was operating during the 2-year period, cases would appear further and further from the original source as time progressed. In both instances, a plot of distance in time vs. geographical distance for all pairs would tend to show a pattern with the points falling around a line from the lower left-hand corner to the upper right-hand corner of the diagram.

In this study, a simple 2×2 analysis was performed by grouping the pairs into those who lived more or less than 250 metres apart, and those who had dates of onset more or less than 14 days apart. The results were as follows:

	≤ 250 m	> 250 m	
≤ 14 days	10	338	348
> 14 days	69	7458	7527
	79	7796	7875

The expected number of cases in the upper left-hand cell would be 79 × 348/7875 = 3.5 (remember the thinking behind χ^2), which is clearly lower than the observed value of 10. The *P*-value was less than 0.005, and this result therefore supports the hypothesis that pityriasis rosea might be transmissible.

Another example of cluster analysis, which this time failed to find any clusters, comes from an early UK government report about the risk of spread of animal-transmissible encephalopathies to humans.[3] This was well before the first diagnosis of human cases of variant Creutzfeldt–Jakob's disease (vCJD), and the study did not address bovine spongiform encephalopathy (BSE) directly, but rather it looked at the data on any association between scrapie in sheep and CJD.

Several human spongiform encephalopathies were known at the time, and at least two of them, namely kuru and CJD, were known to be transmissible. Kuru was discovered in New Guinea, and the route of transmission was shown to be the ceremonial handling and ingestion of human brains infected with the disease. Transmission of CJD was known to occur via neurosurgical instruments, corneal transplants, and injection of human growth hormone extracted from cadaver pituitary glands.

The sheep disease scrapie has been recognized since the eighteenth century, and the reasoning in the report was as follows. If scrapie could be transmitted to humans and appear as CJD or a similar condition, then CJD should be more common in populations living near herds of sheep with a high prevalence of scrapie. In fact, the incidence of CJD is strikingly uniform all over the world. It is a very rare disease with an incidence of about 1 per million population per year. It shows the same incidence in the UK, where scrapie has been endemic for at least 250 years, as in Japan, where scrapie is rare, and Australia, where scrapie is non-existent. A French study at the time had also failed to find any association between local scrapie prevalence and CJD incidence in different regions of France.

This type of meta-analysis or review of a number of published studies provides an interesting philosophical problem, and one which occurs not infrequently in everyday life. The data seem to indicate a lack of transmission of scrapie to humans, but what degree of certainty can we attach to this finding? What is the *P*-value? How high could the risk be and still not be detected in studies such as these? Part of the problem is the lack of a specific hypothesis, such as 'What is the highest risk of transmission of scrapie to humans commensurate with the observed data?'. However, life is full of incomplete answers to imprecise questions, and at some point science will fail us and we must rely on common sense. Just as in clinical medicine, where many of the things we do probably have frail scientific foundations, the control and prevention of infectious diseases in everyday life cannot always stem from impeccable scientific studies, or wait for such studies to be undertaken. There is nothing wrong with relying on common sense so long as one is aware of what one is doing, and one is also ready to rethink in the light of new data.

Since the first cases of vCJD were diagnosed in the UK in 1994 and 1995, it now seems almost certain that animal spongiform encephalopathies can be transmitted to humans. The neuropathological similarities between BSE and vCJD, as well as the numerous experiments in which BSE has been transmitted to other species, provide strong support. Exactly how this transmission occurs is still unclear, and the discovery of a couple of time/space clusters of vCJD in the UK is intriguing.

As a general point about cluster analysis, it should be noted that even if cases of a disease tend to cluster in space and/or time, this does not prove that the disease is infectious. Many other types of exposures could be brief and localized, and would thus also tend to create clusters of cases. In fact, this is probably true of most environmental exposures.

IN SEARCH OF AN INFECTIOUS AETIOLOGY

There exists a long list of diseases for which an infectious aetiology has been postulated. One of the most intensely researched of these is multiple sclerosis, which seems to have some connection with measles, although it is uncertain how. Several studies implicate infection with coxsackie virus as at least one triggering factor in the development of diabetes. Almost everyone believes that some infection lies behind Crohn's disease, and the proposed association between *Chlamydia pneumoniae* and atherosclerosis is receiving much attention. However, for most such diseases with a suspected infectious aetiology the research will be arduous. Long incubation times, low transmission risks and perhaps genetic influences on disease expression are all factors that make the epidemiology of an infection difficult to elucidate.

A special case is provided by the association between infection *in utero* or in childhood and development of disease much later in life. It is well known that some infections during pregnancy, (e.g. rubella, CMV and toxoplasmosis) can have effects that are directly observable at birth, such as malformation or innate infection, but prenatal infection may also be a risk factor for diseases in adolescence or adulthood which are not ordinarily considered to have an infectious aetiology. For example, influenza in the mother has been associated with schizophrenia in adults. One Finnish study looked at the association between viral infections of the central nervous system in childhood and the risk of developing schizophrenia.[4]

This study made use of the type of population registers with unique personal identifiers that have formed the cornerstone of much epidemiological research from the Nordic countries. The original cohort consisted of 96% of all children born in northern Finland during 1966, or 12 058 individuals. At the age of 16 years, 11 017 of these individuals were still alive and residing in Finland, and they formed the study cohort. In 1993 the personal identifiers for all of these young people were matched against the national hospital discharge registry in a search for all diagnoses of psychoses. In total, 76 cases of schizophrenia and 53 other psychoses were found in the cohort.

CNS infections in the cohort were assessed first by looking at the admissions records of the four paediatric hospitals in the area for the period 1966 to 1972 (before the national discharge registry was operational), and then by searching the discharge registry for the period up to 1980, when all of the subjects in the cohort turned 14 years of age. In the study cohort, there were 145 subjects who had had one or more CNS infections.

The 2 × 2 table for this cohort study was as follows:

	Schizophrenia	Total	Risk (%)
CNS infection in childhood	4	145	2.8
No registered CNS infection in childhood	72	10 872	0.66

The relative risk is 2.8/0.66 = 4.2 (95% CI: 1.5–11.3). All four cases in the upper left-hand cell had had viral CNS infections (coxsackie B5 in two cases and adenovirus 7 and mumps in one case each). Their age at infection ranged from 9 days to 7 years. In a subsequent multiple regression analysis which included possible confounders such as paternal social class, gender, perinatal brain damage, and a few others, the adjusted OR was found to be 4.8 (95% CI: 1.65–14).

This risk increase is not negligible, and the results are clearly significant, but my point in the first paragraph of this section is highlighted when you consider that this retrospective cohort study covers 11 017 × 16 = over 176 000 person-years. The search for infectious aetiologies for diseases that are now considered to be non-infectious requires much work.

ECOLOGICAL STUDIES

All of the studies cited so far in this book have focused on individuals. This may seem like a strange statement since, as was stated in the first chapter, epidemiology is about assigning people to different groups. By observing group-defining characteristics of patients, we are trying to see further than the individual patient, in the hope that knowledge of their age, sex, geographical area, behaviour, etc., will aid in diagnosis, treatment and prognosis, and also in the elucidation of risk factors and aetiologies.

However, in all of the previous examples, the exposures and outcomes were measured for individuals. Knowledge of the individual's exposures (where this term is again used in a very general sense, and also includes such factors as gender and age) helps us to assign people to the different groups we want to compare and study. Epidemiology is about comparing groups, but the composition of the groups comes from measurements on individuals.

A different approach is used when entire populations are compared, with little or no knowledge of the individual risk factors and outcomes in those populations. A good example of such an *ecological study* comes from the observation that colon cancer is much more common in Western Europe, where people eat very little fibre, than it is in Central African countries, where people eat plenty of fibre. In such a study, the average fibre intake in two populations is compared, and also the incidence of colon cancer in these two populations. Only the two populations as a whole are studied – we know nothing about the individual fibre intake or the individual risk of colon cancer in the two areas. It could be that those who developed colon cancer in Europe happened to eat as much fibre as the average African, even if the mean European intake was low.

An example of an ecological study that tried to elucidate a possible infectious aetiology for a form of cancer comes from a multicentre project involving 17 populations from 13 different countries.[5]

The bacterium *Helicobacter pylori* was discovered in Australia in the early 1980s. It soon became clear that infection of the stomach wall with this bacterium played a role in the development of gastritis and ulcers. Some studies also indicated an association between infection with *Helicobacter pylori* and cancer of the stomach. In order to clarify this association further, the investigators collected blood samples from around 200 individuals from each of 17 different populations. These people were chosen at random from population-based registers, general practitioners' lists, drivers' licence rosters or health-screening programmes. The aim was to obtain 50 samples each from men and women aged 25–34 and 55–64 years, and subjects who declined to participate were replaced by someone else in the same category with regard to age and sex.

The sera were assayed for antibody to *Helicobacter pylori,* and these results were compared with published national statistics on mortality rates for gastric cancer. The findings of ecological studies are often presented as so-called scatter plots (see Figure 18.1).

A regression line is then fitted to the data and tested for statistical significance as described in Chapter 9. In this study, the values on the x-axis were the proportion of the randomly tested subjects in each population with antibody to *Helicobacter pylori*, and the values on the y-axis were the published death rates from gastric cancer in the corresponding country. The authors found a strongly significant association between these two values, and they

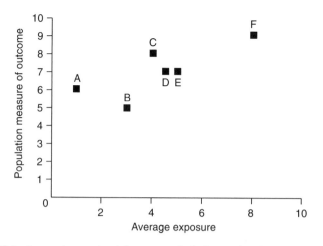

Figure 18.1 Invented example of the way in which the results of an ecological study are usually presented. Each labelled point represents one population, for which an average exposure and an average outcome measure can be assessed.

state that in a population where everyone was infected with *Helicobacter pylori,* there would be a sixfold higher risk of gastric cancer compared with a population where the seroprevalence was zero.

One only has to think about ecological studies for a moment to realize that their major problem is confounding. They compare populations that may differ in many respects apart from the one factor under study. There must be a number of factors that differ between the populations of Central Africa and Western Europe, apart from their intake of fibre.

A somewhat different ecological study, which made clever use of registry data, indicated that some sexually transmitted agent may play a role in the development of cancer of the cervix.[6]

Two data sets were used, namely the yearly notified cases of gonorrhoea in the UK from the mid-1920s to the mid-1970s, and the yearly reported mortality from cervical cancer in women born between 1902 and 1947. Ordinarily, data on cancer incidence or mortality are presented per calendar year, but in this study the author wanted to compare total mortality between age cohorts followed over longer time periods. All women in the UK were therefore grouped into cohorts with the women who were born between 1900 and 1904 in one cohort, those born between 1905 and 1909 in the next, and so on. Mortality from cervical cancer was then only compared between all of the cohorts when the women in each cohort were of the same age (i.e. mortality from cervical cancer in women aged 35–39 years was compared for all of the cohorts, and then mortality in women aged 40–44 years, and so on). Obviously, to be able to perform this calculation one needs data on year of birth for all of the women who died of cervical cancer. The mortality within each cohort was then averaged for all the 5-year intervals along that cohort's life to give a type of mortality rate for that cohort.

Age-specific incidence data for gonorrhoea did not exist for most of the study period, but the author observed that for the years when age was registered, the incidence always seemed to be highest in women aged around 20 years. The assumption was therefore made that each woman was at peak risk of acquiring gonorrhoea at the age of 20 years, and that this risk was equal to the reported overall incidence of gonorrhoea in the year when she turned 20.

For each cohort of women, two curves were plotted on the same diagram. The first was mortality rate for that cohort and the second was reported gonorrhoea incidence at the time when the average age within that cohort was 20 years. The principle is shown in Figure 18.2.

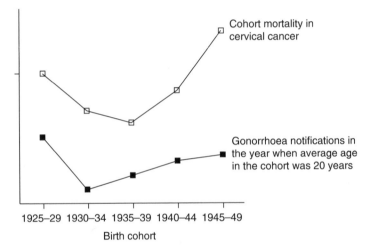

Figure 18.2 Mortality in cervical cancer and national reported gonorrhoea incidence in the year when average age in the cohort was 20 years for five successive cohorts of women in the UK. (*Source:* Beral[6].)

The author demonstrated a correlation between risk of gonorrhoea in young adulthood and subsequent risk of cervical cancer, and since it seemed unlikely that the gonorrhoea infection would be carcinogenic in itself, suggested that it should rather be regarded as a marker for some other unknown sexually transmitted agent which showed the same incidence pattern. Several epidemiological studies have now shown that infection with human papilloma virus is probably the main cause of cervical cancer.

NEWLY DISCOVERED PATHOGENS

The connection between a pathogen and a disease often starts with the discovery of a new pathogen in a number of patients with a common disease pattern. This was the way in which most of the bacteria were coupled to their diseases in the golden era of microbiology at the end of the nineteenth century, when the researchers mentioned in the first paragraph of this chapter were working. A more recent example is given by the bacterium *Helicobacter pylori* mentioned above, and one of its discoverers actually tried to fulfil Koch's postulate by drinking a suspension of the bacteria and observing the symptoms. (He did develop subjective as well as biopsy-proven gastritis.)

Another example comes from the finding of a new organism called coccidian-like or cyanobacterium-like body (CLB) in patients with diarrhoea.[7] The organism was first detected by microscopy in HIV patients, in people with a history of foreign travel, and in a small outbreak at a hospital in Chicago. However, human faeces contain a vast number of microbes, and just because a new one is discovered in diarrhoea patients this does not mean that it is causally associated with the disease. One first step to establish an aetiological role for CLB would be to find an endemic area for the organism and demonstrate that it is more common in people with diarrhoea than in healthy subjects.

This study was conducted among foreign residents and tourists in Nepal. Since 1989, stool samples from such patients with diarrhoea attending either of two outpatient clinics in Kathmandu had been routinely examined for CLB. The number of positive faecal samples had seemed to be highest during the summer months, and it was decided to conduct a prospective case–control study in the summer of 1992.

In order to group subjects into cases and controls, one needs a case definition. The one used here defined diarrhoea as follows:

- a change in the normal pattern of bowel movements; and

- at least three loose stools during a period of 24 hours.

This is quite a common case definition for diarrhoea, but you will find others in the literature.

Controls were chosen from among other attendants at the clinics. They should meet the following criteria:

- no history of diarrhoeal illness during the preceding 2 weeks;

- no history of a CLB infection;

- ability to provide a stool sample.

In previous examples in this book we have just defined the cases, assuming that all individuals who did not meet this definition could be controls. Here the authors also produced a control definition, which is a good idea when the exact spectrum of disease is unknown and one wants to sharpen the distinction between cases and controls as much as possible. CLB was detected in the stools of 108 of 964 patients with diarrhoea (11%), but in only one of 96 control patients (1%). The P-value for this difference can be calculated by the χ^2 method, since the *expected* values for all four cells will be higher than 5, and it was found to be $P = 0.003$.

Next the authors proceeded to look for risk factors for being infected with CLB, and they then conducted another case–control study, in which the cases were now 93 patients diagnosed with CLB infection compared with the 95 CLB-free controls. The groups had similar age and sex distributions, and the proportions of tourists vs. long-term residents were the same. All those 188 people were asked about travel in Nepal during the week prior to the clinic visit, about drinking untreated water, swimming, eating fruit and vegetables, water supplies in their place of residence, etc. Of these variables, only drinking untreated water was significantly associated with infection, for 17 of the 93 cases compared with five of the 94 controls (one control obviously did not answer this question). Water samples from the homes of 22 cases were also analysed, and CLB was found in one of these samples.

When the resident subjects were asked how long they had lived in Nepal, it was found that the median length of stay for the cases was 11 months (inter-quartile range 4–21), but for the controls it was 24 months (range 9–72). The difference was highly significant and could point to some type of immunity to the infection developing with time. In comparisons such as these it is wise to use the median instead of the mean, since just one person with a very long stay would influence the mean disproportionately.

This study therefore shows a strong association between diarrhoea and the finding of CLB in faeces. If one wants to be a purist, there may still be uncertainty about its aetiological role. The organism could still just be a marker of risk if it happened to exist in the environment in the same milieu as the real cause. However, this pathogen should also still be undiscovered, since the CLB cases had the same pattern of other enteric pathogens *(Shigella, Salmonella, Giardia,* etc.) as the healthy controls, and an overall prevalence of any such pathogen less than half of the non-CLB diarrhoea cases.

SUMMARY

Several epidemiological methods exist for investigating whether or not a disease has an infectious aetiology. The basic idea is to look for clusters in time and space which could indicate transmission from infectious to susceptible individuals. If cases show more links than would be expected, or if cases that appear to be close in space also appear to be close in time, there is some evidence for transmission. However, it should be remembered that several environmental exposures will also be localized, so that cases may appear clustered.

For many diseases with a suspected infectious aetiology the demonstration of this fact could be made very difficult by long incubation periods, low transmission risk and a strong influence of other cofactors.

Ecological studies can provide a starting point for clarifying an infectious aetiology, but all such studies have problems with confounding.

The connection of a newly found pathogen to a specific disease pattern is best achieved by fruitful collaboration between the microbiologist and the epidemiologist.

Case–control studies provide a useful tool for elucidating risk factors, which can then be investigated more systematically.

REFERENCES

1. Löffler E. *Mitteilungen aus den Kaiserliche Gesundheitsamt.* Vol. 11, 1884. Translation taken from Brock DT. *Robert Koch. A life in medicine and bacteriology.* Madison, WI: Science Technical Publishers, 1988: 180.

2. Messenger AG, Knox EG, Summerly R, Muston HL, Ilderton E. Case clustering in pityriasis rosea: support for role of an infective agent. *BMJ* 1982; **284:** 371–3.

3. Ministry of Agriculture, Fisheries and Food. *Report of the Working Party on Bovine Spongiform Encephalopathy.* London: HMSO, 1989.

4. Rantakallio P, Jones P, Moring J, von Wendt L. Association between central nervous system infection during childhood and adult-onset schizophrenia and other psychoses: a 28-year follow-up. *Int J Epidemiol* 1997; **26:** 837–43.

5. The Eurogast Study Group. An international association between *Helicobacter pylori* infection and gastric cancer. *Lancet* 1993; **341:** 1359–62.

6. Beral V. Cancer of the cervix: a sexually transmitted infection? *Lancet* 1974; **1:** 1037–40.

7. Hoge CW, Shlim DR, Rajah R et al. Epidemiology of diarrhoeal illness associated with coccidian-like organism among travellers and foreign residents in Nepal. *Lancet* 1993; **341:** 1175–9.

Chapter 19
The epidemiology of vaccination

Here the study of the protection afforded by vaccination is discussed. The concept of vaccine efficacy is introduced, and the difference between direct and indirect effects is explained. The implications of study design of various interpretations of a figure for vaccine efficacy are discussed.

The concept of immunity and the measurement of vaccine-induced immunity are central to infectious disease epidemiology, and really have few counterparts in the study of non-infectious diseases. The fact that some people are resistant to exposures that would always cause disease in others rarely applies to factors such as diet, toxins or radiation. It is true that there may be genetic differences in susceptibility to other harmful exposures, but these are generally poorly understood, and in most instances there is little evidence of the all-or-nothing effect of immunity on susceptibility to infections. The other aspect of vaccine-induced protection that is specific to infectious disease epidemiology is that vaccination, at least in most instances, not only protects the vaccinated subject, but also the people around him or her, in that their exposure to the pathogen will diminish. If enough people in the population are vaccinated, the amount of exposure to the still unvaccinated will decrease to a point where epidemics can no longer be sustained, and we shall have herd immunity in that population, just as discussed in Chapter 11. This concept of *indirect protection* due to other people being vaccinated is important when one wants to measure the effect of a vaccine on individuals, as we shall see below.

VACCINE EFFICACY

The ideal way to measure the protective effect, or *efficacy*, of a vaccine is to perform a regular randomized, controlled clinical trial, in which one group of subjects is given the real vaccine and another group is given placebo. The two halves of the cohort are then followed over time, and the numbers of cases are counted. The incidence rates are calculated for both groups, dividing the number of cases by the number of person-months or person-years in each group.

If the incidence in the vaccinated group is I_v and that in the unvaccinated group is I_u, then the *vaccine efficacy is* defined as follows:

$$VE = \frac{I_u - I_v}{I_u} \times 100 \ (\%)$$

That is, if the vaccine gives total protection there will be no cases at all in the vaccinated group, which means that I_v will be zero, and $VE = I_u/I_u \times 100 = 100\%$. If the vaccine is useless, the incidence will be the same in both groups and VE will be zero.

When vaccine efficacy is assessed in an outbreak situation, the respective attack rates are usually substituted for the incidence rates in the definition of VE.

DIFFERENT TYPES OF STUDIES

A cohort study

One example of a study to measure vaccine efficacy comes from a trial of a *Haemophilus influenzae* type b (HIb) vaccine in the USA.[1]

The entire cohort consisted of 61 080 children who came for a well-care visit to any of 16 centres within a medical care programme in northern California between 1988 and 1990. In order to be included, the children had to have made at least one visit before they were 6 months of age, and infants with known immunodeficiencies were excluded. A complete vaccination consisted of three doses of vaccine during the first year of life. In this study, the subjects were not randomized to receive treatment, and no placebo was used. Children born during the first week of each month were not offered vaccination, and they constituted part of the control group. The rest of the control group consisted of children whose parents were offered vaccination for them but declined.

In order to study the efficacy of a full vaccination, follow-up of vaccinated children to diagnose HIb infections only started 1 week after the third dose. Since the third dose was given at age 8 months on average, an age bias would have been introduced if all of the infections in the control group had been recorded. Therefore follow-up of each control child started when the child was 1 week older than the average age at which the vaccinated children received their third dose. The children in both groups were followed until the age of 18 months. Cases of invasive HIb infection (meningitis, cellulitis, bacteraemia) were detected by several different methods, including weekly reports from nurses at the study centres, monthly listings from the microbiological laboratory of positive HIb cultures from normally sterile sites, discharge notes from hospitals in the area compatible with HIb disease, and requests for reimbursement of hospitalizations outside the area.

In total, 20 800 infants received a full vaccination, and they were compared with 18 862 unvaccinated children who were also followed from the age of 255 days up until 18 months. The numbers of person-years in the two groups were 12 949 and 11 335, respectively. There were 12 cases of severe

HIb disease in the unvaccinated children, compared with none in the vaccinated group. In this case, I_u would therefore be 12/11 335 and I_v would be 0/12 949, and vaccine efficacy would be estimated to be 100%. The confidence interval for this estimate can be calculated using the formula for the confidence interval for zero, described in Chapter 7. There were no cases in the vaccinated group. The upper 95% confidence limit for this value of 0 is 3.7. Using this figure instead of 0 in the formula for VE, we obtain a lower 95% limit for the VE of 68%.

Since this was not a randomized trial, extra care must be taken to exclude possible biases. If for some reason the vaccinated children had been at lower risk of HIb infection than the children in the control group, then the estimated VE would be too high. The report presents a number of indications that this was not the case, the most valid being that the incidence in the control group was no higher than that among all of the children at the participating centres during the years preceding the study, and also lower than the concurrent incidence among the children in the area who were not taking part in the study.

The authors justify the chosen design with two arguments, the first being that it is logistically difficult and time-consuming to undertake a randomized study of this size, and the second argument being that there was an increasing demand for HIb vaccination among the parents in the area during the period. This last argument points to a possible confounder, as with all probability the better educated parents will be the ones who demand vaccination first, and if risk of severe disease is associated with social class, there may have been a lower incidence among the children in the treatment group even in the absence of vaccination.

Several of the large Finnish studies of new vaccines during the 1980s and 1990s have also simplified the randomization process by assigning children born on even or odd dates to either the treatment or placebo group. It is difficult to envisage that this could introduce any bias, but it removes the blinding.

A case–control study

An important theoretical paper published in 1984[2] pointed out the possibility of using a case–control design in attempts to measure vaccine efficacy. This approach was used in a study of meningococcal vaccine in Brazil.[3]

A total of 137 cases of bacteriologically confirmed meningitis with *Neisseria meningitidis* serogroup B occurring in children aged 3 to 83 months were collected in São Paulo during 1990 and 1991. For each child, four controls were selected, matched with regard to age and neighbourhood. The controls were recruited in a very hands-on fashion with the interviewer starting in front of the home of the case and then walking to the first house to the left, and enquiring about children of an appropriate age in the household. The interviewer then continued to call on houses down the street to the end of the block, and if this was not enough to recruit four controls, they returned to the starting point and proceeded to the right along the street. As a last resort, the interviewer went around the entire block in an anticlockwise direction.

In a case–control design, the objective is to assess whether there is any difference between the proportions vaccinated in the case group and the control group. If all cases are unvaccinated and all controls are vaccinated, this would obviously indicate that the vaccine has a protective effect. In this study, the vaccination status of cases and controls was determined solely from vaccination cards given to the mothers at vaccination. All children with an indefinite vaccination status were excluded from the analysis.

Of the original 137 cases, it was not possible to select controls for 10 cases, and for a further 15 cases vaccination status was indefinite. A total of 409 controls had a definite vaccination status, and they were matched to the 112 remaining cases; 68 of the cases (61%) had been vaccinated, compared with 260 of the controls (64%).

If you look back at the above definition of VE, you can see that the formula can be rearranged as follows:

$$VE = \frac{(I_u - I_v)}{I_u} = 1 - \frac{I_v}{I_u} = 1 - RR$$

where RR is the relative risk of disease in vaccinated compared with unvaccinated individuals. An obvious extension of this formula to the case–control situation would be to substitute OR for RR. In this study, the OR for being vaccinated according to disease status can be calculated from the 2×2 table as follows:

	Meningitis	**Control**	
Vaccinated	68	260	328
Not vaccinated	44	149	193
	112	409	521

The OR value becomes $(68 \times 149)/(260 \times 44) = 0.89$, and the estimated vaccine efficacy would thus be $(1 - 0.89) \times 100 = 11\%$. This is not very impressive, but the authors then went on to show that age at vaccination seemed to be very important, and that the VE in children aged over 4 years when they were vaccinated was as high as 73%.

A crucial prerequisite for all non-randomized studies of vaccine efficacy is that there is no difference in exposure between the two groups – vaccination must be completely at random with regards to future risk for disease. A good example of a situation in which an estimate like the one above would be totally misleading comes from the current Swedish strategy for BCG vaccination. General BCG vaccination was abandoned in 1975, and since then the aim has been to offer the vaccine only to children at increased risk of tuberculosis. These are mainly children of immigrants from countries where TB is still much more common than in Sweden. If this selection of higher-risk children could be perfected so as to be totally accurate (i.e. with 100% sensitivity in identifying children who might later be infected with TB) and the vaccine has less than 100% efficacy, then all of the cases of TB in Sweden in the future will appear in vaccinated children. Someone who was ignorant of this bias in vaccination might regard such a finding as an indication of very poor VE.

A somewhat different randomized controlled trial

An alternative study design was used in another trial of meningococcal vaccine, this time in Norway.[5] Instead of randomly allocating vaccine or placebo to individual subjects, the unit of randomization was school. Since meningococcal disease in Norway shows a peak for the age group 13–21 years, it was decided to undertake the study in 1335 secondary schools on pupils who were 14–16 years old. Each school was randomized to receive either vaccine or placebo to give to all of its participating students, and the investigators, school nurses and students were all blind to the content of each school's batch. In total, 74% of all Norwegian pupils in the 14–16 years age group agreed to participate. The vaccine group consisted of 88 000 pupils in 690 schools, and the placebo group consisted of 83 000 students in 645 schools.

A full vaccination consisted of two injections, and cases of meningococcal disease among the participants were only counted if they occurred more than 2 weeks after the second injection. Cases were chiefly ascertained through the well-performing laboratory reporting system that had previously been set up in Norway.

During the study period, there were 89 confirmed cases of group B meningococcal disease in the age group. In total, 63 of these had been pupils of secondary schools, and 39 of these were participants in the study, but one of them had the disease before the study started and two became ill less than 2 weeks after the second injection (both of these pupils were later found to have received placebo). Since the unit of randomization was school, individual cases should not be counted, but rather school outbreaks. However, all cases except two were singular.

There were 11 outbreaks (12 cases) in the 690 vaccine schools compared with 24 outbreaks in the 645 placebo schools. The 'per school incidence' was thus 11/690 = 0.016 vs. 24/645 = 0.037, and the vaccine efficacy measured on a school basis would be VE = 1 – 0.016/0.037 = 57%.

The difference between the two groups of schools can be shown to have a P-value of 0.012 with Fisher's exact test (which was here performed one-sided, since there was no reason to believe that vaccine efficacy would be negative).

The authors conclude that this VE is too low to justify a general vaccination against meningococcal group B infections in Norway, since the yearly incidence is only around 200 cases. A very different conclusion could be drawn from quite similar numerical findings from a study of an oral typhoid vaccine in Indonesia.[5] The estimated VE for this vaccine was also only around 50%, but the incidence of typhoid in the country is so high that 250 000 cases per year could theoretically be prevented by a vaccination programme with good coverage.

Three different ways of estimating VE

In a measles outbreak in Niamey, Niger, in the winter of 1990 to 1991, vaccine efficacy was estimated by three different methods.[6] The study included all children up to the age of 5 years, but we shall only look at those aged 9–11 months here. There were 1199 cases reported in this age group. From a vaccine coverage survey performed just before the outbreak, it was known that coverage in these infants was 63%.

One approximate method for estimating vaccine efficacy is called the *screening method*, which uses the following formula:

$$VE = \frac{PPV - PCV}{PPV(1 - PCV)}$$

where PPV is the proportion of the population vaccinated, and PCV is the proportion of the cases that have been vaccinated (that is, those cases who were not protected by their vaccination).

The log books of the 29 clinics in Niamey were screened for the period of the outbreak for records of vaccination status in the cases. For 142 of the 1199 cases, vaccination status was unclear, but of the remaining 1057 cases, 198 were vaccinated. Assuming that the vaccinated/unvaccinated distribution was similar among those with unknown status, PCV can thus be estimated to be 18.7%.

The screening method gives the estimate of VE as $(0.63 - 0.187)/[0.63(1 - 0.187)] = 0.865$, or 87%.

The investigators also performed a retrospective cohort study in which the selection of households was undertaken in a manner which is quite common in studies in developing countries. From a starting point in the middle of a village or town sector, one chooses a direction completely at random (e.g. by spinning an empty bottle). One then walks to the nearest household in this direction, the occupants are interviewed, and the investigator moves on to the nearest household that has not yet been interviewed, and so on. In this study, four starting points were used and a total of 165 households were interviewed about age, sex, vaccination and disease status of the children. The incidence of measles could then be compared in vaccinated and unvaccinated children.

This type of cohort study raises several interesting questions with regard to the sizes of the unvaccinated and vaccinated groups – the denominators. The outbreak lasted for 7 months, and during this period children moved in and out of the age group 9–11 months. They could also be vaccinated at some time during the outbreak, but were then not counted as vaccinated until 14 days after they had received the vaccine. Finally, they could become ill with measles, and would then leave the cohort. All of this means that the sizes of the two groups that were compared change almost daily, and the researchers actually calculated the number of days as susceptible or as vaccinated for each child in the cohort. There were 1219 person-days contributed by vaccinated children, and 4069 person-days contributed by unvaccinated ones. The numbers of cases in each group were two and nine, respectively. The VE was then calculated using the incidence density instead of incidence in the standard formula. By this method, VE was estimated to be 26%.

The third estimate of VE was made with a case–control study. A total of 250 cases were enrolled at six of the health clinics, and for each case a matched control was selected from children attending the clinic for a different illness. Vaccination status in cases and controls was assessed from the vaccination card. VE was calculated with the formula $VE = 1 - OR$, where the OR is a matched-pair OR (something we have not covered in this book). The VE was estimated to be 89%.

The discrepancy between the cohort study result and the other two results can probably be explained by the fact that there were only 11 cases in total in this age group in the cohort.

DIRECT VS. INDIRECT PROTECTION

The Norwegian study described above is also interesting from another perspective apart from the block randomization, and that has to do with indirect protection. During outbreaks of meningococcal infections there will be a high prevalence of healthy carriers in the population, many times higher than the proportion who actually become ill. In an outbreak in a military camp in Sweden several years ago, meningococci could be isolated from the throats of over 50% of the soldiers. Even during non-epidemic periods, around 5% of young adults in Northern countries are healthy carriers.

As was discussed briefly at the beginning of this chapter, vaccines offer protection not only to the vaccinated in individuals, but also to the people whom they might otherwise have infected. At least this is true if the vaccine protects against infection as well as disease, and in fact many bacterial vaccines also seem to protect against carriage. If this was the case with the vaccine used in the Norwegian study, exposure would have been lower in the vaccine schools than in the placebo schools, since there would have been fewer carriers in the former group. (In fact, the vaccine used in this study seems to have had no effect on carriage, but the reasoning holds true for many other vaccines.) The classic definition of vaccine efficacy assumes that the degree of exposure is similar in the vaccinated and unvaccinated groups, and does not take into account such indirect effects. However, it may well be argued that the figure measured in a study such as this is more interesting from a public health point of view, giving an estimate of the population effect not just of the vaccine, but of an entire vaccination programme. The combined direct and indirect protection of a programme is sometimes referred to as its *effectiveness*.

The implications of different study designs could be demonstrated by the following schematic diagrams. First assume that all subjects within one population (a school, a town, or a country) are vaccinated, whilst another similar population serves as the control group (see Figure 19.1).

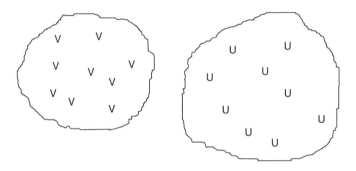

Figure 19.1 A vaccine trial comparing one totally vaccinated (V) and one totally unvaccinated (U) population.

It is quite evident that if the vaccine prevents not only disease but also carriage, then exposure would be lower in the population on the left, and a vaccine efficacy according to the above formula would be an overestimate.

If we instead vaccinate 50% of the subjects in a given population, the situation would be as shown in Figure 19.2.

In this case, at least if vaccinated and unvaccinated individuals mixed freely, exposure to both groups would be the same, and the VE would be

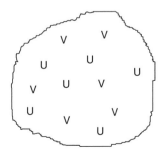

Figure 19.2 A vaccine trial in which vaccinated (V) and unvaccinated (U) individuals can mix freely.

valid. However, you should note that in this situation the exposure of unvaccinated individuals will also decrease (since the prevalence of carriers is also lower), so that the overall incidence will be lower than before the vaccine was introduced. If the study was designed to detect a certain difference in incidence between the groups, one might well find that one obtained fewer cases in the control group than was anticipated on the basis of pre-trial data, and the study findings might not achieve the statistical significance one had hoped for.

ASSESSING EFFECTIVENESS BY SURVEILLANCE

The ultimate method of assessing the overall effectiveness of a large-scale vaccination programme is obviously by observing a clear decrease in the incidence of disease. One nice example of rapid effect comes from the introduction of HIb vaccine in Finland.[7]

The trials of one type of vaccine started in 1986–87 when three doses were offered to 50% of all infants, group allocation being by date of birth. During the period 1988–89, two two-dose vaccines were compared, each being given to 50% of all infants, and since 1990 another type of two-dose vaccine has been offered to all infants. The authors maintain that all cases of HIb meningitis treated in hospital in Helsinki since at least the early 1970s have been recorded, and that fairly reliable data are available back to the late 1940s. The actual age of each of these cases was not known, but from reliable surveillance data from the period 1984–90 they can postulate that 90% of the cases should have been in the 0–4 years age group.

Since the population of the Helsinki area was increasing during this period, the yearly number of cases has to be divided by the actual number of newborn to 4-year-olds in order to obtain comparable incidence figures. The results for four 5-year periods with good data are shown in Table 19.1.

This study may have been performed a little early, since the vaccination programme had hardly started to have any effect in the last 5-year period, but there does seem to be a break in a previously upward trend. Another

Table 19.1 Incidence of *Haemophilus influenzae* type b meningitis in Helsinki during the period from 1946 to 1990 (incidence in children under 5 years of age is estimated) (*Source:* Peltola et al.[7])

Five-year period	Cases Total	Annual	Population of 0 to 4-year-olds	Yearly incidence per 100 000 0 to 4-year-olds*
1946–50	36	7	39 900	16
1966–70	65	13	51 800	23
1976–80	117	23	49 500	43
1986–90	68	14	51 800	24

* Assuming that 90% of all cases were in this age group.

important piece of information in the article is that there was not one case of HIb meningitis in the age group in the Helsinki area in 1991.

Later studies from several countries have shown a rapid decline in invasive HIb disease after the start of a general vaccination programme, and also an indirect effect in that age cohorts which are too old to be included in the newly started programmes have also shown a decreasing incidence.

EVALUATION BY SEROLOGY

As you can see from the above examples from the USA and Norway, modern cohort studies of vaccine efficacy tend to become quite large. This is due to the fact that even if severe HIb and meningococcal infections are important public health problems, the incidence is still low. In the US study, 0.6 unvaccinated children per 1000 had severe infections during the study period, and in the Norwegian study only 0.3 per 1000. Especially if the vaccine efficacy is a little lower than 100%, such incidence figures will necessitate large groups in order to achieve any significant differences. One alternative and quicker approach is to resort to serological methods, and measure the levels of antibody to the vaccine after vaccination. Ideally, the antibody measured should be protective, and not just a marker of seroconversion, and there should also be some defined titre that is known to be protective. The VE would then be estimated as the proportion of a vaccinated group that acquires protective levels of antibody after vaccination.

Such serological methods are often also used to follow the waning effect of a vaccination. In the absence of any natural or man-made boosters, the level of any antibody will decay with time. When the titre falls below the protective level, the vaccination is assumed to be no longer protective, and estimates of the average time from vaccination until loss of protective antibody levels have been used in various vaccination programmes to determine when a booster dose is needed.

In a study of hepatitis B vaccination in The Gambia, 1041 children were recruited into a cohort with the aim of giving everyone at least three injections during the first year of life. The clearly protective level of hepatitis B virus surface antibody (anti-HBs) is usually assumed to be more than 100 international units (IU) per litre (L), whilst a level of less than 10 IU/L is considered to indicate lack of protection. Subjects with anti-HBs values between 10 and 100 IU/L probably have some protection.

The problem with any study of a vaccine that requires more than one dose is to get all of the study subjects fully vaccinated. There will always be those who just had one dose, or two, and the question is how these should be accounted for. In a regular clinical trial of a vaccine, they would most often be excluded, but when one is trying to assess a vaccination programme rather than just the vaccine itself, they should be included. This will give a better estimate of how the vaccine will perform in the more routine health-care situation. In the Gambia study, only 87% of the children had received three or four doses of the vaccine during their first year of life, but the results were analysed for all children who had had at least one dose. At age 1 year, 763 children who had not had a natural hepatitis B infection could be traced and tested for antibody, and of those 92% had a level of over 100 IU/L, 6% between 100 and 10 IU/L, and 2% below 10 IU/L. Serology would thus indicate that the VE was at least 92%, and perhaps as high as 98%.

The mean antibody level decreased by 75% from age 1 to 2 years, and by another 28% from age 2 to 3 years. Such a rapid decline in antibody during the year after the vaccination is seen for most vaccines, but need only cause concern if non-protective levels are reached too soon, and in fact the proportion of unprotected children increased only slightly. At the age of 2 years only 4% had anti-HBs below 10 IU/L, and at the age of 3 years, 5%.

In total, 19 of 698 vaccinated children tested at age 3 years showed serological markers of having had a natural hepatitis B infection, although none of them had demonstrated any clinical signs of hepatitis. Five of these still had an acute or chronic infection with positive HBsAg. However, two of these were probably infected by their mothers at birth, one had a proven and one had a probable post-vaccination level of less than 10 IU/L, and one had a level of 57 IU/L in the first year. The remaining 14 children had just seroconverted in anti-HBc antibody, which showed that they had probably had a natural infection, and several of these had had post-vaccination titres of protection well over 100 IU/L. These results therefore show that one should be careful when assuming that generally accepted protective levels after vaccination always do protect against infection. As with most other laboratory values in medicine, biological variation is important, and the significance of an individual figure may be different for different individuals.

Another study, which indirectly questioned the validity of commonly assumed cut-off values for protective titres, was performed in Sweden to assess the need for booster diphtheria vaccination in children.[9] Diphtheria antitoxin levels were measured in 6-, 10- and 16-year-old children who had been given three doses in infancy. The aim of the study was to determine by how much titres had declined and by how much they could be boosted by an additional shot, but it also provided data on pre-booster protective levels. It was found that the children who had received the three doses at ages 3, 4.5 and 15 months had significantly higher remaining titres than those who had received them at ages 3, 4.5, and 6 months. Of the children who received the more condensed schedule, as many as 48% had titres below the protective level before receiving a booster at the age of 10 years. Another study also showed very low titres in adults. However, at about the same time, in 1984, the first outbreak of diphtheria in Sweden since the late 1950s occurred, with 17 diagnosed cases. Most of the patients were elderly men with alcohol-related problems, and only one case occurred in a child. There was very little evidence of spread to a more general population, even though a high proportion seemed to lack protection, and thus the validity of the cut-off values assumed for protection would seem to be dubious.

WHAT DOES A FIGURE FOR VE MEAN?

The concept of vaccine efficacy as explained above seems quite straightforward, being a measure of how much the incidence (or attack rate) decreases in vaccinated subjects. However, there are two quite different ways of interpreting a figure of, say, 80% efficacy for a certain vaccine:

1. either 80% of the vaccinated subjects obtain total protection against the infection, and the remaining 20% obtain none, or

2. all of the vaccinated subjects show a decrease in their susceptibility to infection of 80%.

Another way of expressing the second alternative is to say that everyone who is vaccinated is protected against 80% of all possible exposures.

In any clinical trial of vaccine efficacy, the difference between these two interpretations becomes very important, but for many commonly used vaccines it is not known which type of protection they confer. The problem concerns the time period for which the vaccinated and unvaccinated groups are followed in the study. If the vaccine is one that gives total protection for a proportion of the vaccinated subjects but none for the rest, it will not matter how long the study runs. The estimated figure for efficacy will tend to be correct in short trials as well as in long ones, even if the precision of the estimate will of course be greater in a longer trial. However, if the vaccine works by increasing the minimum dose of the pathogen needed for infection, this means that just by chance the probability of anyone who is vaccinated encountering a high enough dose to cause infection will increase with time. For such vaccines, the calculated VE will depend on the time period over which the subjects are followed, and it will decrease with the length of the study. Furthermore, estimates of VE will be different in different countries – in a country with high general levels of exposure the efficacy will seem to be lower than in a country with low levels.

This difference in mode of action will also be very relevant when one wants to evaluate how soon booster vaccinations need to be given after a primary immunization. Is a perceived increase in incidence in vaccinated subjects with time due to waning immunity, or is it just a sign of a vaccine effect of type 2 above?

HERD IMMUNITY AND ERADICATION

Discussions about vaccine coverage often utilize the concepts introduced in Chapter 11 on modelling. The most important of these has already been discussed there, namely the relationship between basic reproductive rate and the vaccine coverage necessary for herd immunity. You will remember that the minimum proportion, p, of the population that needs to be immunized in order to obtain herd immunity is given by the following formula:

$$p > 1 - 1/R_0$$

so that the higher the basic reproductive rate, the closer one will have to be to total immunization coverage.

Again, note the difference between the terms 'immunized' and 'vaccinated'. The latter is usually taken to mean those who were injected with the vaccine, whereas the former refers to those in whom the vaccine actually worked. A vaccination coverage of 100% will thus only have an *immunization* coverage equal to the VE of the specific vaccine.

The issue of herd immunity through vaccination is of course intimately linked to the possibility of *eradication* of an infectious disease. If the actual reproductive rate in the population can be kept below 1 for long enough, the disease will eventually vanish. (Obviously this last statement is only true for infections that are spread exclusively between humans. It seems unlikely that diseases such as plague, salmonella, tick-borne encephalitis or tetanus will ever be eradicated.)

Thus considerations of R_0 and maximum vaccine coverage achievable in a programme are very important and real aspects of public health strategy.

Another non-trivial effect of large-scale vaccination programmes is that the average age at infection will be shifted upwards. This also follows from the concepts introduced in Chapter 11. When a high proportion of the population are immune, the risk of a susceptible subject meeting an infectious one will decrease. If every hundredth contact is infectious instead of every teenth one, the average time until one meets an infectious case will obviously increase. This means that diseases which were previously almost exclusively childhood infections will start appearing in adolescents and adults. In some instances, only the *proportion* of cases that appear in adults will increase, whereas the total number of adult infections will decrease, since the overall incidence is falling. However, in other situations there may be a true increase in adult incidence.

One very important example is provided by vaccinations against rubella. The reason for vaccinating children against rubella is not to protect them against an infection which is in fact quite mild in most cases, but to protect women from an infection during pregnancy which may lead to congenital malformations in their child. In the absence of vaccination, the majority of women will have acquired immunity before they reach fertile age, and the objective of a vaccination programme would be to decrease further the proportion of susceptible pregnant women. However, some vaccination schedules might in fact increase this proportion. Consider what happens when the vaccine is first introduced. Usually a programme will start by immunizing all infants born in a certain year, and then successive birth cohorts during the following years. The slightly older siblings will not be vaccinated, but will be subject to reduced exposure from their immunized younger brothers and sisters. Thus there will be an age cohort consisting of the children who were around 1 to 5 years old when the programme started who will reach adolescence with a considerably lower prevalence of immunity than their older or younger siblings.

This very dangerous effect of the programme will eventually disappear about 40 years after the start of the programme (when all women who become pregnant will have been vaccinated), but a continuing uptake below herd immunity level might still increase the number of susceptible pregnant women. Some countries started their rubella vaccine programmes by just immunizing girls at the age of 12 years, but considerations such as the above have led to a change in policy to vaccinate boys and girls. A further consequence of this reasoning is that rubella vaccination programmes should not be started in a country where an uptake corresponding to at least herd immunity level cannot be guaranteed.

SUMMARY

The study of vaccinations is an important branch of infectious disease epidemiology. Vaccine efficacy is defined as the percentage reduction in incidence in vaccinated compared to unvaccinated individuals. However, it does not take into account the reduction in exposure caused by decreasing incidence in vaccinated people close to the study subjects (i.e. the indirect effects of vaccination).

For vaccine studies in which subjects are not randomized to vaccine or placebo, it is crucial that there is no difference in exposure between the two groups. If this can be shown to hold, case–control studies may provide a quicker and easier way to measure vaccine efficacy.

Since vaccine studies that assess actual incidence tend to be large and lengthy projects, an often used alternative is to measure antibody levels in vaccinated subjects. The problem here is being certain of exactly which types of antibodies, and which levels, correspond to protection.

For many vaccines it is unclear whether the figure for efficacy denotes the proportion of vaccinated subjects who will derive total protection, or an overall reduction in susceptibility provided to all of those who are vaccinated. This difference has important implications for the design of studies to measure vaccine efficacy, especially with regard to the length of the study.

With vaccine-maintained herd immunity, it may be possible to eradicate certain infectious diseases. However, large-scale vaccination programmes will shift the age distribution of cases which, especially in the case of rubella, might have serious consequences.

REFERENCES

1. Black SB, Shinefield HR, Fireman B *et al.* Efficacy in infancy of oligosaccharide conjugate *Haemophilus influenzae* type b (HbOC) vaccine in a United States population of 61 080 children. *Pediatr Infect Dis J* 1991; **10:** 97–104.

2. Smith PG, Rodrigues LC, Fine PEM. Assessment of the protective efficacy of vaccines against common diseases using case–control and cohort studies. *Int J Epidemiol* 1984; **13:** 87–93.

3. De Moraes JC, Perkins BA, Camargo MCC *et al.* Protective efficacy of a serogroup B meningococcal vaccine in São Paulo, Brazil. *Lancet* 1992; **340:** 1074–8.

4. Bjune G, Høiby EA, Grønnesby JK *et al.* Effect of outer membrane vesicle vaccine against group B meningococcal disease in Norway. *Lancet* 1991; **338:** 1093–6.

5. Simanjuntak CH, Paleologo FP, Punjabi NH *et al.* Oral immunisation against typhoid fever in Indonesia with Ty21a vaccine. *Lancet* 1991; **338:** 1055–9.

6. Malfait P, Jataou IM, Jollet MC, Margot A, de Benoist AC, Moren A. Measles epidemic in the urban community of Niamey: transmission patterns, vaccine efficacy and immunization strategies, Niger, 1990 to 1991. *Pediatr Infect Dis J* 1994; **13:** 38–45.

7. Peltola H, Kilpi T, Anttila M. Rapid disappearance of *Haemophilus influenzae* type b meningitis after routine childhood immunisation with conjugate vaccines. *Lancet* 1992; **340:** 592–4.

8. Chotard J, Inskip HM, Hall AJ *et al.* The Gambia hepatitis intervention study: follow-up of a cohort of children vaccinated against hepatitis B. *J Infect Dis* 1992; **166:** 764–8.

9. Mark A, Christenson B, Granström M *et al.* Immunity and immunization of children against diphtheria in Sweden. *Eur J Clin Microbiol Infect Dis* 1989; **8:** 214–19.

Chapter 20
The epidemiology of
AIDS and variant CJD

Here many of the methodological problems that were touched upon in the previous chapters are discussed again by reference to examples from the study of the epidemiology of AIDS and variant Creutzfeldt–Jakob's disease.

The last two decades have seen the discovery of two new infectious diseases with complex epidemiology, namely AIDS and variant Creutzfeldt–Jakob's disease (vCJD). The study of these two diseases highlights most of the methodological problems discussed in previous chapters, and this is why I have included this chapter at the end of the book – as a recapitulation.

AIDS

Short background

The new disease 'acquired immunodeficiency syndrome' was first described in 1981, and a system for notification was set up shortly thereafter, first in the USA by the Centers for Disease Control (CDC), and subsequently in other countries. As was highlighted in the discussion of outbreaks in Chapter 12, such surveillance requires a case definition, and the CDC published a list of symptoms and diseases that should define a case of AIDS. This list contained a number of so-called opportunistic infections (i.e. infections with pathogens that do not cause disease in otherwise healthy people) and a number of malignancies. The two most important case-defining conditions were pneumonia caused by the fungus *Pneumocystis carinii* and the vascular skin tumour known as Kaposi's sarcoma.

The first years' surveillance indicated that the disease mainly affected men who had had sexual intercourse with other men, people who had been in contact with Haiti or Africa, and people who had received a blood transfusion. During these years there was much debate about the aetiology of AIDS, and many theories were advanced. One was that semen itself was immunodepressive, especially in anal intercourse, and another was that repeated exposure to many pathogens, mainly the virus CMV, led to exhaustion of the immune system. The study of the association between poppers and AIDS has already been mentioned in Chapter 5.

Although epidemiological research revealed strong risk factors, one could not say that epidemiological science managed to establish that AIDS was an infectious disease. However, in 1984 the human immunodeficiency virus was isolated, and its role in the pathogenesis of AIDS became clear. Tests for antibody to HIV were available for use in the clinic from 1985, and they showed that many people were infected with the virus without showing any symptoms of AIDS. At about the same time it became possible to test for the virus itself in infected people, and the Western blot was introduced. This test analyses the exact pattern of antibody response in seropositive people and makes it possible to determine whether this is a true infection or just a non-specific reaction in the tested person. The polymerase chain reaction (PCR) was first used to test for HIV virus in the late 1980s.

Incidence/prevalence

One of the major problems in AIDS epidemiology has been to gain an idea of the number of people who are infected with HIV in a country, and also to measure the rate of spread of the virus. By the mid-1980s it was clear from clinical follow-up, as well as from HIV tests of stored blood samples, that the time from infection with HIV to the development of AIDS must be several years on average. A notification scheme for AIDS will thus not show the actual incidence of HIV infection in a country, but rather the incidence several years ago.

This is another example of the problem with subclinical infections discussed in Chapter 13 on surveillance. Most people who are infected with HIV will not notice it, and they will not come to a clinic to be diagnosed and notified. About one-third of those who are infected actually do experience an acute viral illness a few weeks after the infection, with fever, sore throat and sometimes a rash, but this is often too mild or non-specific to lead to a diagnosis.

Thus the only certain way to assess the prevalence of HIV infection in a country would be to test a representative sample of the population for HIV antibody. However, ever since the epidemic was first recognized, many people have had a very deep personal anxiety about being found to be seropositive, and members of already stigmatized groups such as homosexual men and injecting drug users have feared registration by the authorities. The number of people who would choose to abstain from such a test would probably be too large to make the result valid. This is especially true for most industrialized countries, where the overall prevalence has been low, and where the result of testing even a large sample would be difficult to interpret if just a few individuals declined to participate.

An alternative strategy is to test people who come into contact with the health-care system, and who are either asked directly to provide a sample for HIV testing, or whose blood is drawn for other tests, but could also be used to look for HIV antibody. (Since most countries now agree that it is unethical to test people for HIV without their knowledge, the latter option requires that all identifying information linking a test result to a person should first be removed from the blood specimen.) Examples of such groups include blood donors, hospital patients in general, and pregnant women. However, there are a number of problems with selection bias for each of these groups.

1. Potential blood donors are explicitly asked about a number of factors and behaviours that correlate with the risk of being HIV positive, and if they admit to these factors or behaviours, they are not allowed to donate blood. This means that there will be an under-representation of people at risk among blood donors. Also, we know little about the characteristics of blood donors compared with the general population.

2. The age distribution of patients in hospital is heavily skewed towards higher ages. Even if blood samples from outpatients were included, the group of men between adolescence and 50 years of age would still be very much under-represented. Young women at least come into contact with the health-care system for reasons concerned with contraception or pregnancy, but men of a similar age may not see a physician for decades. Obviously, sera from patients will also include a disproportionate number of people who are ill for other reasons, and it is not clear how this relates to HIV prevalence.

3. Pregnant women are probably the most representative of these three groups, since around 80–90% of all women have at least one child during their lifetime. Again, however, it is uncertain how the probability of being pregnant relates to the risk of being HIV positive. Consider past infections with sexually transmitted diseases as an example. Such episodes increase the risk that a woman will be infertile, but there is also a positive association between past sexually transmitted infections and the probability of being HIV positive. This means that HIV prevalence may well be higher in those women who do not become pregnant.

All of the above are examples of selection bias, as we discussed in Chapter 6. None of the three groups is entirely representative of the general population, and the HIV prevalence in any of these groups cannot be assumed to be equal to the overall prevalence.

Measuring the *incidence* of HIV infection is even more difficult. The only certain way would be to have reliable yearly estimates of prevalence, and to calculate the changes between them. To achieve this for a representative sample of the population would be very difficult.

Incubation time

Much research has been undertaken during the last two decades to elucidate the natural history of HIV infection, and especially the time between infection with HIV and the development of AIDS. This period has historically been called the incubation time of AIDS, which is of course strictly speaking incorrect. The incubation period should be for the HIV infection, and the time until the development of AIDS should be called the asymptomatic phase or something similar. We do not usually talk about the incubation time to liver cirrhosis in patients with hepatitis C infection, which would be an exact parallel. Acknowledging that this is a misnomer, we shall adhere to ordinary usage here.

One reason for this interest, apart from its obvious relevance to patients and physicians, is that the incubation time is an important variable if one wants to model the HIV epidemic. Since a large proportion of the people who have progressed to AIDS will be too ill to take part in the transmission of the virus, the incubation time would correspond approximately to D, or the duration of infectivity, as discussed in Chapter 11. If one wants to calculate the basic reproductive rate for HIV infection using the following formula:

$$R_0 = \beta \times \kappa \times D,$$

where β is the risk of transmission per contact, κ is the number of contacts per time unit and D is the infectious period (measured in the same time unit as κ), then one must know the value of D.

The first reports on incubation times were based on clinical cohorts, where seropositive patients were followed and the percentage who developed AIDS after 1, 2, 3, etc., years of follow-up were reported. This approach neglects the fact that the patients had been infected for an unknown period of time before they were first seen in the clinic. The situation is summarized in Figure 20.1.

Each line in the figure represents a patient. The left-hand end denotes the actual date of infection (which is usually not known to either the patient or

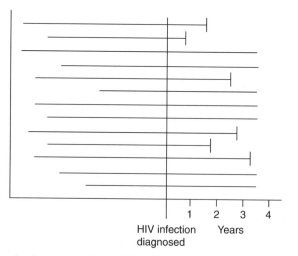

Figure 20.1 A schematic graph of a follow-up study of 13 HIV-positive patients.

the physician). For simplicity, we here assume that all of these 13 patients with HIV infection were diagnosed at the same time, at the beginning of year 1. The vertical bars at the right-hand end of the lines correspond to AIDS diagnosis in a patient.

A description of the rate of AIDS development in this cohort would be that in the first year, one out of 13 patients was diagnosed with AIDS, after 2 years a total of three patients were diagnosed, after 3 years a total of five, etc. These figures would not tell us anything about the real incubation time, since they fail to include the unknown time from infection to diagnosis of HIV positivity.

Estimates of the incubation period for vCJD have exactly the same problems, as we shall see below.

Other studies conducted at around the same time used a method that is also biased, but where this is not so easily detected.[1,2] They recognized the problem with regard to unknown infection dates, and only looked at AIDS cases who had been HIV-infected from a blood transfusion, and for whom the actual day of infection could therefore be ascertained. The average time from transfusion to AIDS diagnosis could be calculated in this group of patients. However, this approach can only be used to investigate individuals who have developed AIDS when the study is conducted. At the same time there are also an unknown number of people infected via blood transfusion who have not yet developed AIDS, and in whom the HIV infection is not even diagnosed. The situation is illustrated in Figure 20.2, where the left-hand end of each line again shows when a patient was infected, and the vertical bars represent AIDS diagnoses.

Here we would know exactly when the four patients who had developed AIDS were infected. The average incubation time for them seems to be about

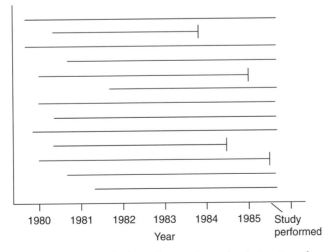

Figure 20.2 A schematic graph of a study reporting on incubation times for transfusion-associated AIDS cases.

4 years. However, the other nine patients would be totally unknown to us, and we could not see that they were still asymptomatic HIV-positive. The method described here will underestimate the true incubation time since, in effect, it will only detect those patients who have short incubation times.

The correct method for measuring the incubation time is obviously to follow a cohort of seropositive individuals with known infection dates. The first such studies were conducted on a cohort of haemophiliacs infected via factor concentrate transfusion recipients,[3] and on a cohort of homosexual men in San Francisco who had stored blood samples from a hepatitis B vaccine trial in the late 1970s, just when HIV started to spread there.[4] The present estimate of the median incubation time to AIDS is around 10 years, but there seems to be a wide range from short periods of just 1–2 years up to 15 years or more in individual patients. The upper limit is still unknown, and studies of the full natural history of HIV infection may never be conducted, since the advent of effective anti-retroviral therapy has (fortunately) distorted the picture.

Transmission routes

Not even the discovery of the three major transmission routes for HIV infection, namely sexual intercourse, blood-to-blood contact, and mother-to-child contact, could really be ascribed to formal epidemiological studies, but rather it is due to growing collective evidence from clinical observations.

Instead, the real role of epidemiology has been to show how HIV is *not* transmitted. It is obviously unethical to expose people to the virus in different ways to see whether or not they acquire the infection, and we must make use of the information provided by the epidemic itself. Important issues in the early years were whether or not HIV could be transmitted in social contacts, such as hugging, kissing or just sharing a glass. The possibility that mosquitoes could transfer the infection was also discussed.

In order to answer the first question, serological studies of family members to known HIV-positive patients were conducted. Those family members had often lived with the patient for a number of years before the infection was diagnosed, and had experienced the full range of social contacts with him or her. No transmission to individuals other than sexual partners was discovered in several hundred household contacts from different countries, which showed that the risk of social transmission must be very low.

With regard to the issue of mosquito-borne infection, early seroprevalence studies from Africa showed that the prevalence was appreciable in infants, practically zero from age 5 years to adolescence, and then rose with increasing age into the twenties. If mosquitoes could transmit HIV, it would be highly unlikely that children were spared. The age pattern seems to be more consistent with transmission from mother to infant, and with a rise at the age when sexual activity begins.

You might suggest that another useful way to discover possible routes of transmission would be to interview known HIV patients about how they might have become infected. This suggestion touches on a general problem with regard to using surveillance data for infectious disease epidemiology. Once a number of transmission routes for a disease have been scientifically established, the physician who diagnoses a case will ask the patient about these specific exposures, and will be satisfied if the patient acknowledges any of them. For HIV surveillance this means that if the patient acknowledges intravenous drug use, then his infection will be ascribed to that transmission route. If he acknowledges that he has had sexual intercourse with another man, his infection will be labelled 'homosexual transmission', and so on. Almost anyone who does not admit to either of these two specific risk behaviours will at least acknowledge engaging in heterosexual intercourse. Since this is a known risk factor, it will be assumed to be the actual route of transmission, and being such a common behaviour it could mask the existence of unknown routes.

Non-sexual transmission

Studies of recipients of blood transfusions from an infected donor have shown that the risk of infection is virtually 100%. These studies usually start with one diagnosed case of HIV infection in a recipient, then go on to find the donor, and finally trace all of his or her other recipients, and could thus be regarded as retrospective cohort studies.

The risk of transmission in the health-care setting, mainly from accidental needlestick injuries, has been assessed in prospective cohort studies. Health-care workers who pricked themselves with a needle that had been used for an HIV-positive patient, or who cut themselves on contaminated glass or other sharp objects, were monitored to see whether they developed antibody to HIV. Obviously the estimated risk would be too high if people who were already infected with HIV when the accident occurred were included in the cohorts, and most studies have stipulated that a so-called baseline blood sample must be taken directly after the accident.

The probability that an HIV-positive pregnant woman will transmit the infection to her child, either during pregnancy or at birth, can also be assessed in prospective cohort studies in which the babies of known positive mothers are followed up after birth.[5] This seems straightforward enough, and I should refrain from going into the real subtleties of HIV epidemiology in this chapter, but I shall point out just one in this context. Who are the mothers whose HIV status is known prior to delivery? Is there anything special about them that could bias the selection of known HIV-positive women? Well, one common reason for being tested is that the woman has previously given birth to a child who developed AIDS. If some women are at greater risk of transmitting HIV, then they would have a higher probability of already being diagnosed. Those women would thus be over-represented in the original cohort, and the sample would not be representative of all HIV-positive pregnant women. Such a selection bias should render the calculated overall transmission risk too high. This example shows that one cannot be too careful when looking for biases. Alternatively, it might be seen as demonstrating that there is a limit to how far one should pursue one's methodological rigour, especially since the last decimal of the calculated risk probably has very little practical relevance.

Sexual transmission

It has proved very difficult to assign exact numbers to the risk of HIV transmission in various situations, and especially to the risk in sexual contacts. Admittedly, it could be argued that exact values are of little practical importance. For example, what difference would it make either to the individual or to public health programmes whether the risk of transmission in vaginal intercourse was 0.1%, 1% or even 10%? Would the exact level of risk really affect the health message? However, for the purpose of modelling the epidemic, these are important figures, corresponding to the variable β in the above formula for the basic reproductive rate.

The main problem when studying sexual transmission is the long incubation time. For most HIV patients it is unknown when or by whom they were infected. Our knowledge of transmission probability comes mainly from the study of couples in which one partner is discovered to be positive. When this partner's date of infection is known, as in transfusion recipients or many haemophiliac men, it becomes possible to calculate the risk per 'couple-year' by testing the other partner and combining a number of such couples in a retrospective cohort study. It must of course be assumed that the other partner could not have become infected by someone else.

Prospective studies of risk of sexual transmission are difficult, since most couples in which one partner is positive and one is negative will change to safer sexual behaviour (e.g. by using condoms more consistently than before). This means that the assessed risk will no longer correspond to the more 'natural' situation in which the two partners' HIV status is unknown to them.

Several couple studies have shown that the risk of transmission increases if the infective partner has developed symptoms of HIV infection. However, such studies have a major problem with confounding. If the infective partner is symptomatic, he or she has probably been infected for a long time, and the couple has probably had sexual intercourse many times. An asymptomatic infective individual may have become infected recently, and will not have exposed his or her partner so many times.

There has been much debate about the role of other STIs in HIV transmission. Does a person who has another STI transmit HIV more readily, and will an HIV-negative person with an STI become infected more easily? This is also an issue where confounding is a problem, as many case–control studies have shown that HIV-positive patients have a higher prevalence of other STIs, or a higher seroprevalence of markers for past such infections, than HIV-negative controls. The problem is that all STIs are acquired in the same manner, and that people whose sexual behaviour puts them at high risk for acquiring gonorrhoea, syphilis, herpes, etc., will be exactly the same individuals who are at risk of becoming infected with HIV.

The best (and most often cited) study of the relationship between STIs and HIV was conducted in the Mwanza Region of Northern Tanzania in the early 1990s.[6] The objective of this study was to determine whether improved STI control would lower the incidence of HIV infection in a randomized trial.

A total of 12 communities defined by a health centre with its surrounding catchment area were selected as elements for randomization. HIV prevalence in the region was known to vary with distance from Lake Victoria, degree of urbanization, and distance from a major road, and communities were matched pair-wise according to these variables. Within each pair of communities, one was then randomized to receive intervention, and the other was not. Intervention consisted of greatly improved STI services and prevention efforts in the health centre of the community, including syndromic diagnosis, safe supply of drugs, health education and free condoms. After the 2-year study period, this intervention was extended to all 12 communities, as to do anything else would have been unethical.

In each community, about 1000 adults were randomly selected into a cohort. They were surveyed at the start of the study and after 2 years, when 71% of the originally included subjects could be contacted. The outcome was as shown in Table 20.1.

The crude RRs were adjusted for age, sex, travel during follow-up, history

Table 20.1 Two-year HIV incidence in matched communities in the Mwanza Region (*Source:* Grosskurth et al.[6])

| Matched pair | HIV seroconversions | | Adjusted RR |
	Intervention (%)	Comparison (%)	
Rural	5/568 (0.9)	10/702 (1.4)	0.59
Islands	4/776 (0.5)	7/833 (0.8)	0.65
Roadside	17/650 (2.6)	20/630 (3.2)	0.88
Lakeshore	13/734 (1.8)	23/760 (3.0)	0.62
Lakeshore	4/732 (0.5)	12/782 (1.5)	0.35
Rural	5/699 (0.7)	10/693 (1.4)	0.50
Overall	48/4149 (1.2)	82/4400 (1.9)	0.58 (95% CI: 0.42–0.79)

of STI (ever) at the start of the cohort, and male circumcision. The overall RR was calculated as the geometric mean of the six individual RRs.

The Norwegian vaccine study described in Chapter 19 used schools as a unit of randomization, and this one used communities. In both cases this means that the statistical analysis is not by individuals. In this study, the sample size is therefore 12. This number had been chosen in order to be able to detect a reduction in annual HIV incidence from 1.0% to 0.5% with 80% power.

The conclusion drawn from the Mwanza study was that the provision of good curative and preventive STI services in a community reduces the HIV incidence by 40%.

Mixing patterns

Mixing patterns obviously play a major role in determining the shape of the AIDS epidemic. They also become important for estimates of the magnitude of different risk factors. Several case–control studies have correlated the risk of HIV infection with the number of sexual partners that the person has had. Others have calculated the odds for infection according to type of sexual contact, (e.g. oral vs. anal intercourse). Most of these studies implicitly assume that exposure remains constant over time, and that it is uniformly distributed across all partners.

Studies of the first type may ascribe an increase in prevalence to a corresponding increase in the average number of partners. However, if the prevalence rises in the studied group, that means that they will also infect their partners to a greater degree, which in turn leads to a higher risk per contact for the study subjects. This interaction between the studied group and their partners is actually quite complex, especially if one wants to analyse the pattern over time. If you recall the example about herpes simplex type 2 infection in pregnant women in Chapter 9, we said that increasing seroprevalence at a certain age over a 20-year period could be due to having a higher number of partners before becoming pregnant. However, it is just as likely that the proportion of all men who were infectious had increased with time, so that the risk per partner had also increased. In fact, since we did observe an increased seroprevalence among the women, this must also have led to an increased prevalence among the men who were their partners. Without corresponding seroprevalence data for men, it becomes impossible to determine which of the two explanations for the increase in women is likely to be more correct.

Of course, the risk of infection associated with different behaviours also depends on the prevalence of infection in the presumptive partners. Suppose that a certain type of sexual behaviour is very common in one group and another type of behaviour is common in another. If HIV, just by chance, is introduced into the former group first, then the behaviour in that group will appear to carry a much higher transmission risk just because the susceptible members of that group will have a higher probability of meeting an infected partner.[7]

Both of these examples are somewhat theoretical, but they point to problems that can be overlooked by epidemiologists who are not used to thinking in terms of infectivity and mixing patterns.

For the modellers, the above discussions imply that we can obtain useful values for β and D, even if we have to use a whole array of different β values for different types of contact. Also, we might have to assume that β increases, for example, when a person is infected with an STI. However, the remaining problem is κ, namely the number of contacts per unit time. If the population were neatly divided into distinct compartments, such as injecting drug users, homosexual men, heterosexual men and women, etc., we could possibly obtain some value of κ for each of them. The problem is that the compartments are not distinct, and we know very little about how often contacts occur between them. The very simple model presented in Chapter 11 does not account for this situation, and it remains a problem even for much more elaborate and complex models.

However, the figures given in this chapter may be used for a simple example of the use of the formula for R_0. There is some support for estimating the attack rate of HIV in a heterosexual relationship to be about 10% (i.e. β). The average time from infection until the development of AIDS seems to be around 10 years (i.e. D). What rate of partner change per year (κ) would be needed in a heterosexual population in order to keep HIV endemic? The formula would be as follows:

$$R_0 = 0.1 \times \kappa \times 10 = \kappa$$

In an endemic situation, $R_0 = 1$, which would give a value for κ of 1. This is the same as to stating that if people changed partners on average every year, then HIV would remain endemic in this population. If the rate of partner change was higher, there would be an epidemic situation.

VARIANT CREUTZFELDT–JAKOB'S DISEASE

Short background

In 1985, the first cases of a previously unknown, deadly disease in cows were diagnosed in the UK. Because of its obvious psychological and neurological symptoms, it was soon named 'mad cow disease'. The epidemic grew exponentially during the latter half of the 1980s, reaching a peak of almost 40 000 cows in 1991 (see Figure 20.3).

Quite early in the epidemic, it was coupled to the feeding to cows of meat- and bonemeal produced from sick or dead animals. The disease was found to

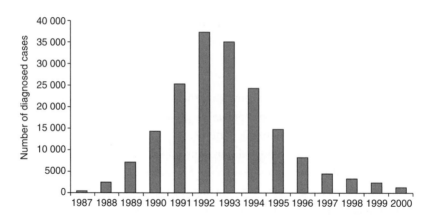

Figure 20.3 Diagnosed cases of bovine spongiform encephalopathy in the UK during the period 1987–2000. Note that the bar for 1987 includes a few cases diagnosed before this period.

belong to the group of transmissible spongiform encephalopathies, of which scrapie is another example, and the scientific name became bovine spongiform encephalopathy (BSE). Cases in other species were also diagnosed, and experiments showed that BSE could be transmitted from the brain of a sick cow to laboratory animals, mainly by direct injection of brain material into their brains, but also via the oral route.

In 1996, 10 cases of a new type of CJD in humans in the UK were first described.[8] This variant form differed from classical CJD in that the patients were much younger, and they had other symptoms, a longer survival, and a different brain tissue pathology. The patients had become ill during 1994 and 1995.

Outbreak analysis

These 10 cases clearly represented an outbreak. What was the source? A case study failed to reveal any common pattern among the patients. They were of both sexes, from different parts of the country, had no profession in common, and shared no other apparent risk factors. However, they had all eaten beef.

To perform a proper case–control study in this situation was very difficult. For one thing, most of the patients had such severe dementia when diagnosed that it was impossible to interview them. Also, as was pointed out in Chapter 5, a case–control study in which one has no clue of what one is looking for is almost always futile. It was known from other prion diseases in humans and in animals that the incubation time is very long, so what exposures would one ask for? Furthermore, since around 80–90% of the population ate beef at the time, the finding that 10 out of 10 patients had this exposure could hardly achieve any statistical significance.

The strongest support for a link between BSE and vCJD was an ecological one. Both epidemics started in the same place at approximately the same time.

Incubation time

The problems in assessing the incubation time of vCJD are the same as those for AIDS in the 1980s. Early in the outbreak we will only have seen the patients with short incubation times. However, we can assume that the first cases in cows appeared in 1984 or 1985, and we know that the dangerous parts of the cow were taken out of food production from around 1990. Since the first human case became ill in 1994, the lower limit of the incubation period must be between 4 and 10 years, but what is the upper limit?

Some clues may be obtained by looking at similar diseases. The disease kuru that was mentioned in Chapter 18 is another transmissible spongiform encephalopathy (TSE) of humans, with an upper limit for the incubation period of several decades. The incubation period for iatrogenic transmission of 'classic' CJD is easy to measure, since the exact date of exposure (dura transplant, growth hormone injection, etc.) is usually known. At the time of writing it is estimated to be between 1.5 and 18 years, but the upper limit is still not certain, as there may be asymptomatic cases who have not yet developed the disease.

Surveillance

Many countries have now set up surveillance systems for vCJD. Since the disease is new and rare, and very few doctors have seen a case, it is very likely that cases would be missed, if there were any. One way to overcome this problem is to increase the sensitivity of the surveillance system by extending it to cover all forms of human TSEs, including classic CJD and a few other extremely rare but similar diseases. The risk that any cases might be missed can be decreased even further if surveillance is not only based on diagnosed cases, but also includes the suspect ones. The ratio between the number of suspect cases reported in the system and the number of CJD cases that are finally confirmed can then be used as a crude measure of the sensitivity of the system. In most of the European countries that are currently engaged in such surveillance, this ratio is about 3 : 1.

The case definition for vCJD builds on a neuropathological examination of the brain for final confirmation. This procedure will not be performed in all patients, which means that at any one stage of the epidemic there will be four groups of cases:

- probable, still alive;

- probable, deceased, awaiting neuropathological confirmation;

- probable, deceased and never confirmed;

- deceased and confirmed.

A constant question for all surveillance systems is what date should be assigned to the cases that are registered and reported. Ideally, it should be the date of onset of disease, as in an epidemic curve, but this is not always known. The second-best option is the date of diagnosis, but for both of these dates reporting delay creates a problem of statistics and sometimes of communicating the data, as recent cases have not yet been reported, and all epidemics thus seem to have turned down during the last reporting period. Since, for any disease, cases diagnosed for example in April will often not be reported until May or June, the monthly incidence reported in early May will show a rather low number for April. Similarly, the annual total number of cases diagnosed last year will always be too low if presented in January, and will be corrected upwards during the following months. This is why most routine surveillance systems publish their data by date of report, as this figure is fixed, and it will not be changed later by delays. In a series of annual reports, this will mean that cases diagnosed late in 1999 will appear in the year 2000 total, but also that some of the year 2000 cases will appear in the 2001 total. This artefact will thus even out if the variations in incidence are not too great.

In an evolving epidemic, the carry-over from one year to the next will not even be approximately constant, and reporting by date of onset or of diagnosis will always display the apparent recent decrease in incidence described above. The epidemic curve usually shown for cases of vCJD in the UK is thus based on year of death in confirmed cases, and those were the data for the curve in Figure 3.2 back in Chapter 3. To this curve should be added seven patients, mostly from the early years, who had probable vCJD while still alive, but who were never autopsied.

Another problem with surveillance that was touched upon in Chapter 13 is the increased level of observation brought about by new knowledge and attentiveness. How can we know that there were not any vCJD cases before 1994? And how much of the epidemic curve is explained by improved diagnosis? Some indication that there may have been earlier cases, but that they were misclassified, is given by the data in Table 20.2, which shows all of the reported cases of human TSEs in the UK from 1990 onward.

Note that Gertsmann–Straussler–Scheinker syndrome, or GSS, is an exceedingly rare TSE.

As can be seen from Table 20.2, the numbers of cases of the three diseases, namely iatrogenic CJD, familial CJD and GSS, have been going down slightly since vCJD was first described. It is possible that there was some previous misclassification here.

Table 20.2 Reported annual deaths from all human transmissible spongiform encephalopathies in the UK during the period 1990–2000 (*Source:* www.doh.gov.uk/cjd/stats accessed on 19 February 2001)

Year	Sporadic CJD	Iatrogenic CJD	Familial CJD	GSS	Confirmed vCJD	Total
1990	28	5	0	0	—	33
1991	32	1	3	0	—	36
1992	43	2	5	1	—	51
1993	38	4	2	2	—	46
1994	51	1	4	3	—	59
1995	35	4	2	3	3	47
1996	40	4	2	4	10	60
1997	59	6	4	1	10	80
1998	63	3	4	1	18	89
1999	61	6	2	0	15	84
2000	39	1	2	0	26	70

Risk of transmission

The major political issue at the time of writing this chapter is the risk of transmission from a cow with BSE. This risk cannot be calculated, since we have no denominator. We are not even 100% certain of the transmission route. What infectious parts have entered the food chain, in what quantities, and how many people have been exposed?

We cannot even be sure of the numerator in the risk calculation, since the incubation period is unknown. How many people will develop the disease? There have been numerous attempts to extrapolate the curve in Figure 3.2, yielding estimates of the final size of the epidemic ranging from a couple of hundred cases to several hundred thousands. However, in this situation, one person's guess is as good as anyone else's. What is clear is that the slope of the increase during the first 6 years is less steep in people than in cows, but this is only as expected when two incubation time distributions are combined.

Transmission routes

Just as for AIDS, epidemiology has so far done little to clarify transmission routes for vCJD. However, the outbreak of this new disease has sparked interest in discovering hitherto unknown routes for classical, sporadic CJD. One case–control study from Australia compared past history of surgical procedures in cases of sporadic CJD with controls.[9]

This study used the Australian National CJD Registry to extract 151 definite and 90 probable cases of CJD reported between 1970 and 1997. Controls were interviewed by means of a random dialling telephone survey. For the cases, medical history, especially past surgical interventions, was assessed mainly from medical records, with information from relatives added, whilst the medical history of the controls was only assessed by means of interviews with relatives.

The types of surgery that were found to be significantly associated with CJD are listed in Table 20.3.

Table 20.3 Association between different surgical procedures and CJD in a register-based case–control study in Australia (*Source*: Collins et al.[9])

Type of surgery	Cases	Controls	OR (95% CI)
Heart	11	19	3.55 (1.57–8.04)
Hysterectomy	28	58	2.96 (1.68–5.21)
Haemorrhoids	8	11	4.46 (1.69–11.8)
Gall-bladder	18	51	2.16 (1.14–4.09)
Hernia	18	46	2.40 (1.26–4.57)
Cataract/eye	24	24	6.13 (3.16–11.9)
Varicose veins	10	15	4.09 (1.71–9.76)
Carpal tunnel	6	4	9.20 (2.48–34.1)

There were also a number of procedures for which no significant association was found (e.g. appendectomy, hip/knee surgery and skin lesions). However, the different methods for collecting information about cases and controls may have led to a bias in this study. This is perhaps indicated by the fact that some minor operations, (e.g. haemorrhoids and varicose veins) showed a significant association. One might believe that these operations would not be so readily communicated to relatives, and would thus appear in the medical records of the cases only.

Another study involved a systematic review of published case–control studies on the association between sporadic CJD and past blood transfusion.[10] This book has not covered meta-analysis, but I shall include this one just as an example.

Systematic reviews of published studies always begin by defining the criteria that these studies must fulfil to be included. In this case, the two criteria were that the studies must

- have studied patients with CJD and controls; and

- have determined the rate of blood transfusion in CJD patients and controls.

Five such studies were identified, published between 1982 and 1999. They ranged in size from 163 to 919 subjects, and the odds ratios for the exposure 'blood transfusion' ranged from 0.54 to 0.89. Only in one did the 95% confidence interval not include 1. The combined OR was 0.70 (95% CI: 0.54–0.89), but one should always be careful about combining data from observational studies.

This systematic review thus indicated a protective effect on the risk of CJD from having received a blood transfusion. The authors point to one potential bias. In three of the five studies, medical or neurological patients were used as controls, and someone who is already a patient probably has a higher probability of having had a blood transfusion in the past. This choice of controls would therefore overestimate this exposure in the background population.

It should also be noted that these two studies only address the transmission of sporadic CJD. We do not know if they apply to vCJD.

SUMMARY

The study of the epidemiology of HIV infection and variant Creutzfeldt–Jakob's disease provides a good list of examples of the problems associated with epidemiology in general. For both diseases, the long, asymptomatic incubation period makes surveillance difficult.

The incubation time distribution can be studied in cohorts, but it is difficult to assemble unbiased cohorts of patients with known infection dates.

With regard to transmission routes, the main achievements of epidemiology have been to clarify how the diseases are *not* transmitted. Also, since almost all cases have been exposed to at least one acknowledged transmission route (heterosexual contact in the one disease and eating meat in the other), routine surveillance has little power to detect additional routes, if these exist.

For HIV:

- strategies to assess prevalence are influenced by selection biases;

- risk of transmission is also best assessed in different types of cohort studies;

- studies of cofactors for transmission, such as stage of infection or concurrent STIs, have problems with confounding;

- mixing patterns influence calculations of risks and odds in ways that are seldom a problem for the epidemiology of non-infectious diseases.

For vCJD:

- modelling is not of much help in predicting the future course of the epidemic;

- the calculation of transmission risk awaits figures for both the numerator and the denominator.

REFERENCES

1. Lui KJ, Lawrence DN, Morgan WM, Peterman TA, Haverkos HW, Bregman DJ. A model-based approach for estimating the mean incubation period of

transfusion-associated acquired immunodeficiency syndrome. *Proc Natl Acad Sci USA* 1986; **83:** 3051–5.

2. Medley GF, Anderson RM, Cox DR, Billard L. Incubation period of AIDS in patients infected via blood transfusion. *Nature* 1987; **328:** 719–21.

3. Giesecke J, Scalia-Tomba GP, Berglund O, Berntorp E, Schulman S, Stigendal L. Incidence of symptoms and AIDS in 146 Swedish haemophiliacs and blood transfusion recipients infected with human immunodeficiency virus. *Br Med J* 1988; **297:** 99–102.

4. Bacchetti P, Moss AR. Incubation period of AIDS in San Francisco. *Nature* 1989; **338:** 251–3.

5. European Collaborative Study. Risk factors for mother-to-child transmission of HIV-1. *Lancet* 1992; **339:** 1007–12.

6. Grosskurth H, Mosha F, Todd J *et al.* Impact of improved treatment of sexually transmitted diseases on HIV infection in rural Tanzania: randomised controlled trial. *Lancet* 1995; **346:** 530–6.

7. Jacquez JA, Simon CP, Koopman J, Sattenspiel L, Percy T. Modelling and analyzing HIV transmission: the effect of contact patterns. *Math Biosci* 1988; **92:** 119–99.

8. Will RG, Ironside JW, Zeidler M *et al.* A new variant of Creutzfeldt–Jakob disease in the UK. *Lancet* 1996; **347:** 921–5.

9. Collins S, Law MG, Fletcher A, Boyd A, Kaldor J, Masters CL. Surgical treatment and risk of sporadic Creutzfeldt–Jakob's disease: a case–control study. *Lancet* 1999; **353:** 693–7.

10. Wilson K, Code C, Ricketts MN. Risk of acquiring Creutzfeldt–Jakob's disease from blood transfusions: systematic review of case–control studies. *BMJ* 2000; **321:** 17–19.

Chapter 21
Further reading

This short chapter lists some books that I have found useful and enjoyable.

There are a large number of books on medical statistics, and it is difficult to mention one above the others. One that I like is *Practical Statistics for Medical Research* by Douglas G Altman, published by Chapman & Hall, London, in 1991.

If you want to learn much more about epidemiology in general, and especially to absorb more about modern thinking and philosophy, you should read *Modern Epidemiology* by Kenneth Rothman, published by Little, Brown and Company, Boston in 1986. There is a new edition (published in 1998) of this book edited by Kenneth Rothman and Sander Greenland, which is excellent but very large. Start with the previous edition.

The best book on the history of infectious diseases, and the one which got me into this field is *Plagues and Peoples* by William H McNeill, published by Penguin Books, Harmondsworth, in 1998.

If you want to learn everything there is to know about field epidemiology, you should read *Field Epidemiology*, edited by Michael Gregg, Richard Dicke and Richard Goodman, and published by Oxford University Press in 1996. This is a very good complement to the book you have just read.

For the francophone, there is a very thorough book on field epidemiology, with a strong theoretical backbone, entitled *Epidémiologie d'intervention*, by François Dabis, Jacques Drucker and Alain Moren, published by Arnette, Paris in 1995.

For those who want to study infectious disease epidemiology in developing countries, a very practical guide is *Methods for Field Trials of Interventions against Tropical Diseases* (second edition), edited by Peter Smith and Richard Morrow, and published by the World Health Organization, Geneva, in 1996.

If you are interested in following news about outbreaks all around the globe, you should subscribe (free) to the electronic discussion forum ProMED. The home page can be found at *www.promedmail.org*.

Index

Page numbers in *italics* refer to figures.